TO JAINE *

STAY ACTIVE... EAT 'CLEAN' FOODS...
AND GOOD THINGS WILL HAPPEN

Michael W.   APRIL 2021

* THANKS FOR MAKING ME A BETTER ATHLETE!

STORMING THE CASTLE

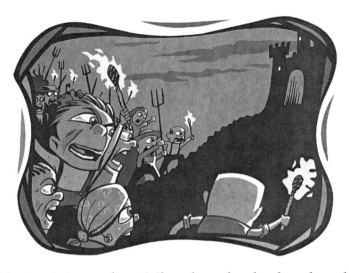

This time it is not the privileged royalty that has abused its position of power, but the massive

FAST FOOD – PROCESSED FOOD INDUSTRIAL COMPLEX

They have fed us cake – and gotten us addicted to other refined non-foods – for too long, resulting in a national and international obesity crisis of unheard-of proportions, while amassing huge profits at the expense of our health. In this Diet Revolution nobody has to wield pitchforks and torches to kill and destroy. Instead, the goal is for us to force them to change their ways: armed with the nutritional knowledge you will gain from reading this book you can change your eating habits and choke off their lifeline – your hard-earned cash – and bring about meaningful change: making wholesome foods of high nutritional value *affordable and widely available*, without cheap, unhealthy flavor enhancers that get us addicted to highly advertised, yet inferior, over-processed, food-like products. The government won't do it for us – our 'public servants' are deep in the pockets of the castle's owners – so we must fight this battle with our feet and our pocketbooks. We have the power to make it happen and break the addiction: for our health, for the health of our children and grandchildren and for a better food supply system in the future.

Diet Revolution Now

Michael Waldau

First published by Dog Ear Publishing
4010 W. 86th Street, Ste H
Indianapolis, IN 46268
www.dogearpublishing.net

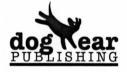

dog ear
PUBLISHING

ISBN: 978-145750-845-5

This book is printed on acid-free paper.

Printed in the United States of America

Table of Contents

HOW SERIOUS IS THE SITUATION?

Dead serious

It's not just about YOU anymore, and losing those 'love handles'. It's potentially much more serious. Consider this FACT: Male offspring of fathers who overate significantly as young adults or in childhood, *even just for a few months*, have a high risk of dying <u>decades</u> sooner than previous generations. The same holds true for female offspring of mothers, so obesity is not "just" a one-time killer anymore - as if this weren't bad enough. It can <u>keep killing</u> for generations to come. And yes, it can happen to <u>you</u>!

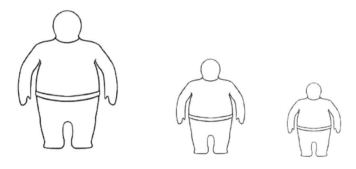

If we do not get the current overweight / obesity crisis under control, obesity in America (and many other industrialized countries) will be so deeply ingrained it will be nearly impossible to avoid reaching epidemic levels. This comes at a staggering cost to our physical and financial well-being, not to mention our healthcare system. We are well on our way: over ¼ of children's calories now come from junk food! And we think nothing of having golden arches franchises in children's hospitals!

Where is the outcry?

What we need NOW is a return to a healthy lifestyle and sound weight management by choosing basic, natural foods that not only taste good, but are also good for us, and by following a more active lifestyle. We have to "re-connect" with real foods – those from which the multinational fast food and industrial food manufacturers have so successfully weaned us. We have to reject the nutritional status quo, overcome a lack of knowledge, and change established habits that have not served us well.

It is time to start our own, individual DIET – and lifestyle - REVOLUTION for ourselves, our children and grandchildren and for the future of a healthy human race.

HI! My name is Michael Waldau

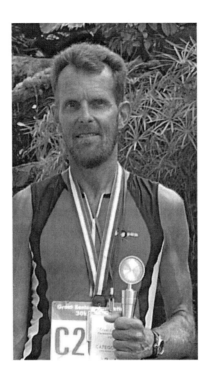

I am not a food scientist
I am not a government nutrition expert at the USDA
I am not a registered dietician
I have never won (or entered) a "biggest loser" competition

So why is this a good thing – and why am I writing a book on nutrition & weight management?

It may be good because of what you are **not** getting:

- You did **not** get the – based on scientific research - **low fat / high carb diet** from me, which started the current obesity crisis in earnest.
- I have also **not** dreamed up the – now discredited - **high protein – low carb diet** either (also backed by sound 'scientific evidence').

- I also can **not** claim to have come up with the grapefruit diet, the hallelujah diet, eat-more-weigh-less diet, weight loss pills, or any number of here-today-discredited-tomorrow diet fads, all claiming to be scientifically proven, and quite often supported by real doctors in photo-op-appropriate lab garb.

- I did **not** have any input into any of the USDA (or other) food pyramids as the cornerstone of a healthy diet. Not the one that never distinguished between refined grains and whole grains (!), good fats or bad fats (!), and that was a thinly veiled advertorial for the dairy and cattle industries. And I cannot claim responsibility for any of the subsequent food pyramid reincarnations or variations that have tinkered with details, were careful not to upset the status quo, but never got to the core of the problems. **My "Food Ark"™ will**, however.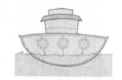

- I am **not** in the pocket of any food manufacturing entity, lobby or restaurant chain, and I do not benefit financially from the current (sad) state of affairs of the nutritional system in this country. The few brand-names I mention / recommend are included without the knowledge of the companies involved, and are based on my personal experience. And – unlike many scientists, government experts, or RDs I do not hesitate to tell you which products (and companies) to choose or to avoid – they don't butter <u>my</u> (gluten-free) bread.

- I do **not** offer "scientifically proven" sensational diet advice ("lose 30 lbs. in 30 days – eating all the foods you want – without exercising!"), or promise other quick fixes. No well-meaning status-quo conventional wisdom here either, which is usually too general, and never goes far enough to address the real issues. No repetitive-to-the-point-of-boredom (and in the end ineffective) yawners here.

- You will **not** find minor (cosmetic) "tweaks" to an existing broken system that will not get you the results you need. "You get out of it what you put into it", and I will not dispense a band-aid approach to deep-seated problems, yet I will not preach "zero tolerance" / "zero compromise" principles.

- And you will **not** find any information about weight-loss surgery in this book!

However you **will** get:

- The hard facts – unencumbered by corporate interests, food lobby–"influenced" advice, or concerns about the effects of nutritional truths on the bottom line of food-for-profit companies.
- "Field tested", tried-and-proven advice from somebody who kept his body fat content in the 5% range for 20-plus years.
- "Real life" advice as to what works and what doesn't for getting your weight in the healthy range, for improving your health through proper nutrition and for making other healthy lifestyle choices.
- The benefit of the experience gained from having been an ACE-certified **Lifestyle & Weight Mgmt Consultant** since 1997, and from having completed numerous diet, nutrition and exercise courses to keep abreast of the latest nutritional developments.

You can rest assured that my suggestions for sometimes *revolutionary* changes in your eating and lifestyle habits are also backed by sound nutritional principles.

WHY I AM WRITING THIS BOOK

There is a lot of misinformation and confusion out there: conflicting health claims, sometimes contradictory dietary advice, misleading advertising, and ever-changing scientific studies, proving, then disproving nutritional theories. Sadly this overload of nutrition-related information (the good, the bad, and the ugly), rather than resulting in a well-informed public, has the opposite effect and results in a dangerous "it's all bad for you" defeatist attitude.

I feel that despite all the information available in various forms and from various sources, ranging from authoritative to quackery, what is lacking is a user-friendly blueprint to a healthier lifestyle. A blueprint that is easy to understand and can be implemented by anyone who is serious about wanting to make a meaningful change in their life, a blueprint that **will** get results.

My goal is to convince people, one book at a time, that **sound nutrition does matter**, that food has a profound impact on quality and quantity of life, and that they **will** notice the difference eating the right foods and making the right lifestyle choices. Eating to survive is not good enough if we **fail to thrive**.

I will call my endeavor a success if there is at least one person who, after reading this book and following the advice given, truly feels that his or her health and quality of life has improved dramatically, and going back to the "bad old ways" is irrevocably out of the question.

But mainly I am writing this book …

BECAUSE NOBODY ELSE IS WRITING THIS KIND OF BOOK!

Oh sure, there is no shortage of well-meaning dietary advice out there. When reading some of it one can just about **hear** the chirpy voices telling us to "eat our vegetables", giving advice on how to "eat less-unhealthy at your friendly neighborhood burger emporium", and advising us to "exercise lightly in 10-minute segments to see glorious results". I don't even want to mention scams that promise miracle weight loss results "without dieting" and "without exercising". You'll also find some generic health statements that the reader has trouble staying awake reading, formulas to estimate your caloric requirements and expenditures (wild guestimates all around), and an assortment of "recent research findings" that are thinly disguised infomercials for certain food products and sometimes paid by same. **You need harder hitting information than that** – preferably from somebody who offers leadership by example, somebody who has kept his weight rock-steady for over 20 years, has had athletic success far beyond the traditional "prime years" by following his own dietary advice, proper training, and keeping his body fat in the 5% range. Somebody who has become immune to temptations by less-than-healthy offerings from giant food processing conglomerates. And above all, you need information from somebody who doesn't have ties to any interest group in the food or diet business.

Certainly **the US Government** is not capable of writing this book. There are too many corporate bottom lines they need to protect; they are too timid to "do the right thing" and let the chips fall where they may; too much an enabler of a corrupt food supply system that needs to be kept in power like a corrupt dictator in a "friendly" nation. Too many subsidized food crops result in a glut of cheap, inferior products. If you don't think that our "Public Servants" are deep in the pockets of various fast-food / processed-food industrial complex companies, think of what would happen to any elected official who came out against any specific food – like beef or dairy, for a (purely hypothetical …) example. The affected industry group would have the senator's lunch – and make sure he won't lunch on the taxpayer's dime after the next elections. Never mind "Remember the Alamo" – **remember 1977** instead. That's when straight-talk recommendations of **reducing** the intake of red meat and dairy products were watered down to suggesting to "choose meats, poultry and fish that will reduce saturated fat intake". And since we all want to reduce those evil saturated fats the implied message is to **increase** consumption of those meats, dairy products and fish that will reduce saturated fat intake (which pretty much leaves only fish on your dinner plate, no?). Clever – and it took 33 years of deceiving the American public for the government to make another attempt at addressing the problem head-on, with the latest recommendations to "eat only moderate amounts of lean meats, poultry and eggs". I would not expect the respective industry groups to shake in their boots and only offer such protein choices, since they know full well that well-meaning but bland recommendations by Big Daddy (aka The Government) are no match for their huge advertising budgets which declare their products (mostly un-changed) "healthy" choices for an active lifestyle. No doubt we'll hear about omega-3 fatty acids mixed into the same deplorable animal feed that will – like a magic wand – turn their offerings into health foods.

The same holds true for other, hardly revolutionary advice emanating from Big G: "Get more of your food from plants" (the new "eat your vegetables", and just as effective), "eat more fish" (yet 2 servings of fish per week is a bit anemic – compared to coming out with a statement that says "*replace* red meat and poultry with fish 3-5 times per week"), "switch to low-fat dairy" (which just confirms a trend that was market-driven for many years), "reduce intake of added sugars and solid fats" (despite the fact that we don't eat "added sugars and solid fats" – we eat donuts and pancakes with corn syrup and melted butter, but Big G wouldn't want to name names), and "reduce sodium and refined grains". Here we go again - heaven forbid we should say the "**d**"-word – **d**onuts, or similar pastries, muffins, breads, crackers, etc. – that could hurt business. "Jobs will be lost" would be the politically correct code words our elected officials would intone.

Bottom Line: Don't expect *real* help and *real* solutions from the government. Consider this: Even in the face of universal agreement in the medical community that fast foods are one of the main culprits of declining health and expanding waistlines, costing taxpayers billions and wrecking whatever health care system we have now or will have in the future, the government is unwilling to do what it should do to any product proven unsafe and hazardous to your health – regulate it. We manage just fine pulling children's toys from the market if infants choke on them. If a product "merely" leads to obesity and diabetes and cardiovascular disease for the majority of Americans (and budget-wrecking healthcare costs) our elected public servants quietly accept campaign contributions from the processed food / fast food industrial complex and wax about the free enterprise system and the individual's right to choose. And we are not even getting close to the really 'big picture' here: consider the fact that in developed countries with the greatest income disparities obesity rates are the highest – and that the U.S. is probably the most obese nation in that category. Do you have any say or control over this? Not by a long shot – but <u>you</u> can make the right decisions about <u>your</u> individual health and counter any and all healthcare trends. The information in this book will help you make those right decisions.

Sadly, also don't expect this book to be written by otherwise highly respected institutions, who all seem to publish their own food pyramids. You might find questionable advice there. Some of their food pyramids allow "Unlimited Amounts" of vegetables and fruit. What did they think the term "unlimited" would mean to nutrition-challenged, obsessive over-eaters? That's right – it's O.K. to eat enough of these foods to get nauseated, or at least seriously overload on fiber and / or sugar, or both, at the expense of a balanced intake of all vital foods.

Also, "75 cal. of sweets" (max) are allowed. So, the term "sweets' encompasses things like … donuts and candy bars and ice cream? Or do they refer to organic home-baked cookies? And do they include Middle Eastern desserts, many of which consist mainly of nuts and honey? How about chocolate? Where are the specifics? How hard could it have been to state instead "75 cal from refined sugars maximum" (which is still 75 calories too many)? Some food pyramids allocate 3-5 servings of fats & oils. What kind of fat might you ask? Duck fat or avocado oil, hydrogenated oils or nuts? Pork rinds or flax seed oil? It appears not to matter. Horrors!

Scientists would seem to be uniquely qualified to write this kind of book. Think again. Yes, everything we know about nutrition & health–related topics, directly or indirectly, we owe to scientific research. The problem there is that their research has become so specialized, that **they** see the Sistine Chapel ceiling paintings one square inch at a time (and can tell you all about it), but **you** want to see the whole picture. Then there is the issue of distilling useful information from lengthy and complicated published findings. For example, applying the knowledge gained from studies of familial hypercholesterolemia in childhood sitosterol and sitostanol can be tricky. And it may not be readily obvious how knowing about thermodynamic and molecular determinants of sterol solubilities in bile salt micelles will improve the quality of your life anytime soon.

Then there is scientific "breakthrough" research suggesting that the super food-du-jour (or a new supplement distilled from it) may help alleviate this-that-or-another condition: Was it a randomized, placebo-controlled, double-blind clinical trial with a large number of participants? Or, was it a one-time study of a handful of test subjects loosely described as "overweight females", "trained athletes" or "older adults with a history of high blood pressure"? Also, has information been divulged about <u>who paid</u> for the latest highly publicized particular study? You might be excused for being skeptical of the findings of a study that seems to prove that you will reap impressive health benefits from eating hunza berries if you found out that the study was funded in whole by the East-Himalayan Hunza Growers Cooperative.

Similarly, it has been said that one can prove just about anything one wants to prove with the properly designed (scientific) study. Have you ever noticed that much of "scientific nutritional research" always seems to prove what the objective of the research or test was? Amazing, no? Add the sheer volume of scientific research data flooding the media with often-times contradictory findings (scientists have egos too ...) and it's no wonder that so many Americans throw up their arms in despair ("enough already"!) and lose interest in staying up-to-date on nutrition and health subjects, or adhering to sound nutritional principles that have stood the test of time. "Everything is bad for me. I might as well have the double cheeseburger - and super-size those fries while you are at it".

How about **doctors** and the medical establishment? Their efforts have made invaluable contributions to a better understanding of health, nutrition and lifestyle choices. But they have also given us liposuction, gastric bypass procedures, miracle weight loss pills, cosmetic surgeries, and endorsed a bewildering array of powerful drugs that sometimes do more harm than good. Too many $-conflicts of interests, and not-always obvious links to pharmaceutical companies, unnecessary procedures, and recommending surgeries as a first resort. Tainted.

So why don't **Registered Dieticians** write this kind of book? They are probably your best bet for personalized nutritional advice, which holds especially true for special population groups. Still, "eat this (relatively healthy in comparison) thing, not that (even worse) thing" advice, generic recommendations (we know already that we should eat our vegetables) and boring "meal planners" with inadequate variety (O.J., oatmeal and low-fat yoghurt for breakfast anyone?) quite often leave you unprepared to make smart 'think on your feet' or long-term decisions for yourself. (Come to think of it, that's not necessarily a bad thing if you are in the diet-advice business). Who can count calories, fat grams and watch for that perfect protein-fat-carbohydrate ratio day-in, day-out? And how much good would it do anyway, knowing that these numbers are educated guesses at best?

To a certain extent RDs can be accused of being part of a failed system that doesn't tread on controversial grounds and they will rarely advocate a bold new approach to the way we eat. And for the life of me I don't understand the elevation of skinless chicken or turkey breast to the status of "cure-all-societal-ills" <u>health food</u>, considering that these parts have grown so big in commercial poultry that the poor birds can't even walk normally anymore! "Do you want a side of growth hormones and antibiotics with that sandwich?"

The question that begs to be asked is where are the role models among the above mentioned groups? How many of these experts (and, giving credit where credit is due, many of them truly are) "walk the talk?" How many of them truly practice what they preach ("eat right") and red-line their respective engines on a regular basis to experience for themselves the theories that they preach? Preciously few.

So, I suggest you expand your search for role models. Go watch a 5K or 10K or similar running race and take a good, hard look at the top finishers in the 50 and over age groups. You'll find some incredibly fit "mature" adults who have stood the test of time and are heads and shoulders above their sedentary age-group compadres. You'll find 60-year olds who can break 20 minutes in a 5K, 50-year olds who run sub-3 hour marathons, or perform similar feats in competitive swimming, cycling, even pole-vaulting, or any other number of sports. The effects of a lifetime of maintaining your weight and staying active aren't so readily obvious with young people in the prime of their lives, when many of them get away with less-than-ideal lifestyle choices. However, once you have reached "mature" territory your past sins, or lack of taking care of your body, cannot be hidden behind well-tailored suits and dresses anymore, much less in a bathing suit. Take a look, and maybe talk to some of these 'over-looked' role models. There are many more out there than you'd think. Some of them may offer dietary advice just like I attempt in this book. Do your research and if you find trustworthy information from other, maybe more educated sources, read it. I do not claim to know it all, be the smartest, fastest, strongest, or the foremost authority on any nutrition or exercise – related subject. I do know however, that this book can be your starting point - or another building block - in your never-ending education on nutrition and health matters.

WHY WE NEED A DIET REVOLUTION

Obesity and being overweight have become the ***standard*** in this country, not the exception anymore. Fully 2/3 of Americans fall into this category, with devastating consequences for their health and our collective pocket books. Think of annual obesity-related costs of $168 **B**illion (and rising) in the United States alone. The added cost obesity adds to an individual's medical bills is estimated to be $2,800.00 p. year! Alarmingly, research has shown that this pattern of being overweight or obese is likely to become deeply ingrained in future generations.

*Serious overeating in childhood or as a young adult (even for periods of time less than a year) can affect our genes and predispose the children of overweight people to **decades** shorter lifespans.*

And this epigenetic "switch" can affect even the offspring of their children, and possibly for generations to come.

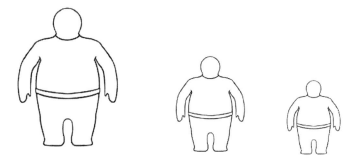

(This "hereditary" effect seems to be passed on from males to male offspring and from females to female offspring only, which is of little consolation to future parents who cannot pick the sex of their children.)

The future doesn't look good, unless we act <u>soon</u> to break this deadly cycle. Americans have tried all the diets known to mankind (and more are on the way) and spent **b**illions of dollars in the process. What do we have to show for it? A <u>healthy</u> diet industry – and a <u>sick</u> and overweight population. Clearly something isn't working here, and quick fixes, minor tweaks, or reliance on cookie-cutter nutritional advice will not fix this mess. No, it's time we did something about it:

Start our very own, personal Diet Revolution

For one, it's NOT all your fault, so stop blaming yourself and get off that guilt trip!

Consider this: some of the brightest minds in the country spend millions of their companies' dollars engineering designed-to-addict foods, throw many more millions into targeted advertising, and make those poor-at-best, empty-calorie-foods at worst, available to you 24/7 wherever you go, at bargain prices. "Real" food has been marginalized, and the odds are heavily stacked against you being able to make healthy food choices. My goal is to arm you to the point where you become immune to temptations of the mighty *fast-food / processed-food industrial complex* by re-learning what <u>real</u> food is all about, what you really need for optimum health, and how to make informed decisions about your lifestyle. Oh, and fall in love with wholesome food in the process, to the point where a sugar-bomb donut or a cholesterol burger no longer have mind-controlling power over you. (I have not had either for decades, and have zero cravings for them.)

More bad news to consider, and not necessarily your fault either: you may be consuming chemicals that make you fat. Far-fetched? Maybe not. Endocrine-disrupting chemicals (EDCs) can mess with your weight-regulating system and promote obesity. They are often called a somewhat catchier, but descriptive term – **obesogens**, and can be found in pesticides (check high pesticide load produce in the Food Ranking Spreadsheet), commercial beef and other meats (grain-fed, and raised in the Big Indoors), unfiltered tap water, and many plastics that get in contact with food. Avoid plastic-wrapped meats, storing or heating or micro-waving food in plastic containers, washing plastic ware in the dishwasher, and in general eliminate as many plastic items that come in contact with your food as possible.

O.K. – I said it is not **all** your fault, but there is enough blame to go around, and you might as well shoulder part of it. <u>I can help you with that part.</u> How? I have been in your shoes, and I know what works, and what is so much smoke-and-mirrors. I couldn't have competed at running races and triathlons for the last 20-some years without that knowledge, and the power to apply it. I didn't do it with yo-yo dieting, quick-loss diets, or magic diet pills. I kept my weight in the perfect range for all those years not by adhering to a rigorous workout regime* (although that helped) that most people can't maintain for long, but by incorporating my knowledge into a **systematic strategy**. Trust me - <u>keeping one's body fat range in the 5% range for over 2 decades is a lot harder than losing any amount of **excess** body weight</u> – sometimes temporarily only. (Sorry, no biggest-loser credentials on my 'resume'.) Additionally I gained invaluable knowledge about nutritional and physical activity issues by becoming an ACE-certified Lifestyle and Weight Management Consultant in 1997 and by staying abreast of the latest scientific findings in the fields of nutrition and exercising.

SO *WHAT'S IN IT FOR* YOU IF YOU START YOUR VERY OWN DIET REVOLUTION?

Whether you want to 'lean up' for the racing season and lose those extra 5 lbs. that will give you an edge, or you want to lose 20, 50, or more pounds, this book can help you make the meaningful changes required to become a fitter, healthier "you". And if all you want to achieve is improving your eating and other lifestyle habits, but don't know how, this book can show you the way.

1. If you feel that your diet and lifestyle are by and large healthy but would like to pick up helpful hints on how to lose a few pounds, this book will do just that for you. Pick and choose what you feel will result in slimming down, and if that doesn't work adopt some of the other strategies in this book. Eventually you **will** succeed.

2. If all you want is eating healthier but aren't sure where to start, you'll find plenty of suggestions. Go "all the way", or <u>change one thing at a time</u>, or gradually make changes, and watch how they improve the quality of your life. I have had the best success when trying a new approach, or eliminating certain poor food choices, by trying it "for just a week" to see what would happen. Invariably I liked how I felt having made

that positive change so much that it was easy never to go back to the "bad old ways", and my new habit stuck. Most people cannot (and maybe should not) toss all their old habits overboard all at once and start over, but gradually make changes that stick. Think of it as a journey, rather than a destination.

3.   If you are overweight to the point of your health – and self-esteem – being affected, your best bet is to follow the advice given in this book to the letter. **You get out of it what you put into it** and you cannot afford half-baked measures. You may want to introduce change gradually, so your system gets used to the good changes you are making. If you were to go from all processed, low-fiber fast foods to all-healthy, high-fiber natural foods overnight, your stomach might not be as cooperative as it would be if you follow the "one step at a time" approach. Ultimately however, you will achieve the best results if you adopt all the measures discussed in this book, and make use of the diet "aids" that come with it. Think of it as a recipe - you can only make so many recipe substitutions and changes before the planned seared ahi tuna with field greens salad turns into canned tuna on iceberg lettuce. And if you have any serious health conditions you should check with your doctor before implementing any drastic changes.

Apart from the nutritional information and mental strategies you can employ, the most important diet "aids" – the one you must use if your goal is meaningful change (all "level 3" folks, per above), are the scale, the scale placemat and a timing device.

- The scale – placemat: you must get into the mindset that regaining control of your life and achieving a healthy weight are the number one priorities in your life. First off you need a good quality scale that consistently shows the correct weight if you step on it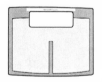
repeatedly. You may not have stepped on a scale in years, but you better start NOW. No need to tell anyone, and seeing that outlandish high number may be additional motivation to "get serious", but you have to establish a base line – call it "Square One". Sure, your long-term goal may be to lose 20, 30, 50

pounds or more, but you can't achieve that overnight. Instead you have to aim for steady, small weight reductions. For example, if you weigh in at 200 lbs. that first time (always first thing in the morning, after your first morning bathroom visit and without clothes) your goal for the next day is obvious: weigh in at 199 lbs. the next morning. Write that magic number (199, in this case) on the placemat with the special pen provided (it wipes off easily with a wet cloth) and use it as your meal placemat for every meal of the day (unless that would prove awkward at work, in which case just use it 'as appropriate'). The goal is that you never, for that whole day, lose sight of your all-important goal – losing that one pound. Every calorie you consume that day has to be weighed carefully (in your mind, not on a real scale) as to whether it will help your goal (to get healthy, necessary food into your system) or jeopardize it (if it is more than you need). Feeling squeamish about displaying your weight to anybody, including your spouse? Fair enough, so just pencil in "XXX – (minus) 1", and only <u>you</u> know what "XXX" stands for. Or add or subtract any number you choose to your current number (weight), so it is only meaningful to you, and not potentially embarrassing.

Why use a placemat? The desire (and need) to lose weight is always on your mind, right? Maybe so, but it's really easy to forget about it during a good meal with friends or family (and even eating alone!) when you might keep eating beyond what you really need. Seeing tomorrow's goal on the placemat during critical mealtimes will make it that much easier to focus on the task and to stop eating when you have had enough. You can then look forward to "good [scale] news" the next morning – *and* a healthy breakfast, preferably after a brisk walk, or a serious workout.

Let's assume you do really well that first day and you meet – or exceed – that goal. Congratulations!!! Celebrate that small victory - and set your goal for the next day for a pound less than this morning's weight. If you don't succeed and your weight remains the same (or goes up – horrors!) don't get discouraged and "dial in" (with removable ink pen) tomorrow's new target – one pound less than today's weight. <u>Be prepared for setbacks!</u> There is no way that you can lose one pound or more every day for any length of time! But aiming for that goal may prevent you from <u>gaining</u> weight. You may stay at a weight plateau, and occasionally you will see increases. Don't despair, re-group, and "stay with the program". Keep in mind that you are not a machine, and weight loss will not happen in a steady, linear manner, but that there will be ups and downs. Also, your body weight can fluctuate greatly from one day to the next – I have experienced gains and losses on the magnitude of 5 lbs. overnight – roughly 3% of my body weight! No need to panic, just go back to "doing the right things" (as outlined in this book), keep weighing in every morning regardless, use the scale placemat religiously, and enjoy those success mornings! They **will** come, once you make the mental "switch". <u>This is critical:</u> serious weight loss starts in your brain, when you throw that switch and want to lose weight more than eating the most tempting food, because you know how it will make you feel once you had too much of it. Don't let yourself go there.

- A timing device, such as an egg-cooker, Timex™ watch, alarm clock, etc.: use it whenever you feel a desire for seconds, "just one more" taste, sweet treat, or must (?) have anything else after a properly sized meal. Promise yourself delayed gratification, set your watch and wait until time is up – THEN revisit the additional food temptation. **This is critical!** This method will not forcibly remove you from the kitchen or the buffet – you'd have to hire me full-time as your personal "food guardian" to accomplish that (you can't afford it …). But, listening to your body 25 minutes after your meal you should hear a loud and clear "full" message, and the desire to have anything else will have evaporated. It works, but like so many things in life (quitting smoking, for one) <u>you have to want it to work</u>. If you want to prove (?) that you still "want" something else, I am sure you can polish off that pint of ice cream – but there shouldn't be an honest craving or desire. Still hungry after time's up? Doubtful, but you may just be plain thirsty, so down a glass of water or fruit tea, etc., and that will fill you up, even though I do not recommend drinking so soon after a meal. Call it the lesser evil. Bottom Line: believe in the power of the 25 minute delay, have small meals, and use a timer of some sort after every meal – it will be your ticket for your slim self to come out, and it **will** work.

---

*Time to explode a myth here: "If you exercise a lot you can eat whatever you want". No you can't, sorry. And you can't eat as *much* as you want either. Bad dietary choices (in quality or quantity) will still catch up with you and result in weight gain and/or poor health. Being fit and slim doesn't guarantee being healthy, so skip those burgers and beers after your next 13.1 race. The good news: chances are you won't have the desire to eat "all you want", because you know how it makes you feel – right then and there, for hours to come, and when it's time to get active again.

SO WHAT'S WRONG WITH CONVENTIONAL NUTRITIONAL ADVICE?

- "Eat **more** vegetables". We've heard it for a long time now - from our mothers, from well-meaning diet experts, weight loss gurus, the U.S. government, and on and on. Yup, 3-5 servings (a nebulous concept for many).
- "Eat **more** fruit" and "eat a greater selection of fruit". Heard that too. 2-4 servings a day. Orange fruit, and purple, white, red, etc.
- "Americans should eat **more** whole grains". It's the foundation of most food pyramids, so there should be lots of it in everybody's diet. Up to 11 servings!
- "Americans don't consume enough fish to benefit from heart-healthy omega 3 fatty acids". Fats and oils are usually 'evil-doers', but there are some 'good guys' in there as well. Like olive oil and fatty fish – if it works for those crafty, long-living Greeks, it must work for us too. Mediterranean diet, here we come! So don't forget - eat **more** fish.
- "The typical American diet is too low in fiber". We have sucked out all untidy non-white ingredients in grains, bleached what doesn't conform, made dazzling-white sugar out of black molasses, removed the brown bran to arrive at sparkling white rice, filtered out all the ungainly looking murky things floating in fresh fruit juice, and on, and on. So yes, by all means, we should consume **more** fiber.
- "Milk is good for you". To suggest otherwise is downright unpatriotic, so drink up! How else are we going to get our calcium and help granny avoid osteoporosis? Cheese and yoghurt are superfoods! Eat **more** dairy products is *the dairy lobby–scripted mantra.*
- As a nation, we should also eat **more** organic foods, **more** high quality proteins such as white chicken or turkey meat, lean red meat, and **more** healthy legumes.

- Oh, and in case you missed all that, you can't help noticing slick advertising on TV or radio or the web or in the grocery aisles exhorting you to eat (**MORE**, of course) this, that or another (processed) food that will help you slim down, lower your cholesterol, be heart-healthy, strengthen your bones or help ward off cancers. There you go again – EAT **MORE** for better health – and even EAT **MORE** to lose weight, and EAT **MORE** pizza to live longer. (I am not making this up.) The list goes on.

All (or mostly) good advice you say? It seems so, but the "read-between-the-lines" message that gets ingrained into our brains once all the other details are long forgotten, is the simple message that we should **EAT MORE,** for weight loss (?) and good health. It's subtle, yet the "**more**" part of the message has its negative effects, regardless of how true each statement may be for many of us. If you think that is an exaggeration, remember the "eat more carbs" (and low-fat) chorus that was nearly impossible to tune out in the 80-ies. Collectively we did just that – ate **more** (highly refined – but low-fat carbs) – without eating **less** of anything else to make up for it, laying the foundation for today's obesity crises.

Here is a fundamental, yet difficult to embrace principle:

Too much of even the healthiest food is bad for your body

ANY FOOD, no matter how wholesome and wonderful it might be in normal quantities as part of a balanced diet, when eaten in excess will be poorly absorbed, and the surplus calories will be stored as fat and will act like a toxic waste site in your body. (Cancers, for one, love toxic waste sites, and fat cells are hungry creatures and want to be fed!) And of course this "too much" of one food will crowd out some of the other foods that are part of a balanced diet. Do you have too much fat stored? Consider this: 2-4% is thought to be "essential" (women get a little slack here: 10-12% is essential, although very athletic females check in lower than that), so chances are excellent that you do. Of course that "essential" range should not be the goal for the vast majority of

Americans, but up to (and no more than) **20%** for men (**25%** for women) would be achievable – and result in huge improvements. Not sure what your body fat percentage is? Have it checked at a "Y" near you, see a healthcare professional, or have it measured in a doctor's office. It's the single best indicator if you are in a healthy weight range. Again, don't worry about the numbers – they are yours to keep secret, but you should know them <u>now</u> ("square one") then track them periodically to gauge your progress.

Back to that **"more"** thinking - it has become all-pervasive in our culture. Just think of super-sized meals that used to be normal sized even one generation ago, from burgers to fries to pies and pop tarts and juice and just about everything else. Or soft drinks, loaded with sugar, or worse yet, high fructose corn syrup. A serving of 12oz does enough damage to your body already (170 empty calories, not to mention all the other unhealthy baggage that comes with it), but nowadays 20oz bottles have become the new standard, and there are 24oz cans out there. Fast-food restaurants serve humongous 32oz or even larger sugar bombs (44oz anyone?) to go with their super-sized burgers and fries. But even nutrition-knowledgeable people can easily fall into the trap of overeating good-for-you foods. Trust me - being overweight from over-eating heart-healthy, lean, organic foods still makes you an unhealthy overweight person. Consider this for a moment: how many obese centenarians do you know? Or 90-year old folks? Octogenarians? Think about that for a moment.

We need to make the switch from "eating more" to "eating less", or **"strategic non-eating"**, to find that perfect balance of minimum calories needed for attaining and maintaining good health. Think of your food intake as a **"just-in-time" inventory system**, without any surplus to put into (toxic) storage for a later famine that – luckily – never comes in most people's lives in this country. Severe calorie-restriction diets may work for longevity and better health, but there is no need for such a dramatic (traumatic?) strategy, as long as we cover caloric requirements for optimum health and constant energy levels – and no more.

IF EATING *MORE* IS NOT THE ANSWER, WHAT IS?

**You guessed it: eating LESS – that is, less of everything.
"Strategic non-eating" I like to call it.
More specifically, put fewer calories from <u>real</u> food into your system than you remove from highly processed foods – and give your body complete non-eating breaks between meals.**

It's as simple as that – and a whole lot more complicated (or else, everybody would do it). For one, since total calories should be reduced for better health (assuming you are overweight, there are no eating disorders or other health issues to contend with) getting the most [nutritional] "bang for your buck" becomes vitally more important. So what foods should we eat less of? Before going into details, let's take a look at the debate raging over "good foods" vs. "bad foods".

It used to be there were clearly defined groups of food. The latest conventional wisdom (or is it a case of being "politically correct" to the manufactures of junk foods?) now declares that there are no "bad" foods. Even foods not known for adding a single healthy calorie to the human diet can be part of a healthy diet, so as not to let cravings develop that will eventually force us to eat a whole box of donuts vs. just one, (sensible?) little donut. So "bad" food can actually be "good" for you, since a little bit of "bad" will keep you from eating a whole lot more of "bad".

I don't buy it. Are fatty pork ribs relatively healthy, considering how much worse pork cracklings are? Is an empty-calorie muffin relatively healthy compared to a smaller empty-calorie cupcake with sugar frosting? And does a donut, deep-fried in heart-healthy, high omega-3 oil, now deserve a government health claim? There's a lot of twisted logic there. I agree that an occasional splurge on "forbidden fruit" does the soul good (lightning will not strike you), but it doesn't make the offending food any better. Here's my list of foods you can – and should – live without:

- **Refined sugar in general, and <u>soft drinks</u> in particular:** loaded with empty calories (TEN or more teaspoons of sugar in <u>one</u> can?!) that don't register with many consumers since they are in liquid form (yes, they 'count'). They often contain phosphoric acid on top of citric acid which speeds up the tooth-decaying effect of sugar and are combined with carbonation – not known for any positive health effects. Carbonated soft drinks - one would be hard pressed to invent a less unhealthy source of calories. Add caffeine to the mix (a proven addictive drug) and one has to wonder why these drinks don't come with a government warning. They will, one day but don't wait for that to happen. Go cold turkey on them now, or gradually reduce your intake, with a concrete total elimination date. Yes, there will be withdrawal symptoms (caffeine <u>and</u> sugar) – which should serve as a scary warning in itself, but you'll feel so much better once you kick the habit, and your body will thank you.
Diet soft drinks are marginally better, assuming they do not contain phosphoric acid, sodium, aspartame, and caffeine. But they are still galaxies away from being in contention to be called "healthy". All highly processed foods should be avoided as much as possible ("all of it" would be a good target), and that holds especially true if you see these ingredients prominently displayed near the top of the list: sugar, corn syrup, HFCS (high fructose corn syrup), glucose, fructose, lactose, dextrose.
- **Donuts:** Over-refined empty calories deep fried in oil of questionable quality (keep in mind how cheap donuts are and draw your conclusions), with boatloads of tooth-decaying simple sugars – how did this ever slip into our "food" supply chain? And you get ignorance-is-bliss bonus points if you buy them in the (usually busy) drive-thru lane of your friendly neighborhood donut shop. Include similar over-processed-to-the-point-of-unrecognizable-to-the-human-body sugar – or fat - bombs so prevalent on supermarket shelves and convenience stores. You know the culprits.

- **High fructose corn syrup (HFCS):** meet one of the food industry's worst inventions ever, even after trying to re-brand itself as "corn sugar". Subsidized by our clairvoyant government and therefore dirt-cheap, it makes for a great flavor enhancer (did I mention *cheap?*), and can be added to a dizzying variety of drinks, juices, and foods you'd never suspect needed it. Empty calories that are not only unnatural and unhealthy but also addictive – and used by your friendly neighborhood food processor to do just that – addict you to their inferior products disguised as foods. Time to read ingredient labels, and when you see them anywhere on the ingredient list, just say no. Better yet – load up on foods that don't need ingredient lists – like vegetables, fruit, quality proteins, nuts, legumes, etc.
- **All 'white flour' products:** "Just say no" to any food that has refined flour as its main ingredient. This includes 90% or more of the so-called "bread' in supermarket aisles, designer (-priced) muffins, 'white' pizza crusts, 'M.I.-Burger' buns, crackers, trendy bagels (super-sized of course), dinner rolls, "healthy" pasta, and such. They form the broad base of not only certain food pyramids (!), but also fertile ground for many "civilization diseases" such as obesity, high blood pressure, adult-onset diabetes, cancers, and many others.
- **Alcohol:** ah, yes, alcohol has recently hired a good P.R. agent, and all of a sudden the fermented red grape juice that only a generation ago was blamed for cirrhoses of French livers has now been elevated to "health food". *"Studies have shown that moderate consumption of red wine can improve your heart health"* we hear a lot. Well, let's look at the small print too, which never makes it onto the label.

It <u>may</u> improve your health -
…"IF your total cholesterol is 200 or higher
… <u>and</u> IF you have a family history of coronary heart disease
… <u>and</u> IF you are 40 years or older
… <u>and</u> IF you smoke

... <u>and</u> IF you have diabetes

... <u>and</u> IF you have hypertension

..." then MAYBE you can reduce your M.I. risk (by a modest amount). Adding up all those "IFs" narrows the number of Americans who could benefit from imbibing to ... what, six? I think it is safe to say that you are a lot better off by going for a 3-mile run in the morning, and including some 'dolmas' (rice wrapped in grape leaves) and fish in your diet, drinking an occasional glass of red grape juice, or just eating grapes (organic, or at least domestically grown). That way you avoid all the baggage of empty alcohol calories (<u>7 per gram</u>), sulfites, additives, potential addiction, headaches, etc., etc.

Granted, an occasional glass of wine may not have an adverse effect on one's longevity or reduction of quality of life, so by all means enjoy that occasional glass, but don't <u>*start*</u> drinking for "health" reasons. As for the other alcoholic beverages out there, like beer and hard liquor, at least they don't pretend to be what they aren't (for good reasons), so let your conscience (and health concerns) be your guide. In short, alcohol just carries too much unhealthy "baggage" with its thin claim to healthful properties to be considered a healthy addition to one's diet.

- **Hydrogenated Fats / Trans Fats:** margarine, the scientists' answer to deadly animal fats, turned out to be deadlier than the product it replaced (butter). This was certainly a scientific Waterloo, although it proved only a temporary setback, as more 'scientifically-backed' – and later repudiated - nutritional advice followed. Just like HFCS, trans-fats are hidden in many processed foods and include some advertising to be wholesome and "natural". You have read the news reports. Transfats promote cancer, heart disease, suppress your immune system, are a big factor in our obesity crisis, and can even mess with reproductive health. And that's not even a complete list of KNOWN health issues, much less the yet-to-be-discovered ones. And yes, these diseases <u>can</u> happen to <u>you</u>.

Again, it pays to read ingredient lists - disqualify any grocery item that contains <u>any</u> of these fats.

- **High sodium foods:** while a little (pure sea salt) is good for most, a lot (of sodium) can be deadly. Americans worry about the evil salt shaker on the dinner table, yet have no reservations downing drinks loaded with sodium, or consuming processed foods that can send their blood pressure into cardiac arrest territory. <u>Sodium can be a killer when consumed in excess, period.</u> Reading ingredient lists and rejecting high sodium foods can be a death-defying act. And since it is a cheap flavor enhancer you wouldn't be surprised that it is prominent in junk food, fast-food restaurant meals, and numerous foods from cheeses to meat products to cereals to sauces to most canned foods.

There you have it – the Killer Triple Threat of high sodium, refined sugars, and "bad" fat – the Processed Food Industry's best friends - with alcohol and refined flour products thrown in for good measure. All of them contribute more than their fair share to the health and obesity crises. Combined, this "Gang of Five" has to shoulder the biggest part of the blame for causing preventable diseases and deaths associated with lifestyle–influenced risk factors in America. Nicotine, lack of physical activity, pollution, and stress are some of the other culprits.

Incredibly, the fast-food / processed food industrial complex spends millions of research dollars to find ever-new ways to use these very same ingredients (did I mention *'cheap'*?) to get us **addicted** to engineered, food-like products that will improve their profit picture at the expense of your health. Why is that? Well, for starters, the food business is a for-profit business. That's not necessarily a bad thing (although there are better alternatives) – just think of the system that was practiced in Eastern Europe under communism. This current for-profit food business, like any other business, feels that gross sales and profits have to grow at a steady rate, if only to please shareholders, not to mention satisfy plain old greed. There isn't a lot of money to be made selling broccoli, potatoes, brown rice, or other "un-sexy" staples in the quantities required for health.

Also keep in mind that the United States would have to be considered a "mature food market". There are approx. 300 million mouths to feed, and that number inches up rather slowly over years, certainly not at growth rates that big corporations – and shareholders - like to see. These 300 million people only **need** so many calories for a healthy existence (and they are trying hard to do their part for the economy by consuming a lot more than that), and in general are only willing to spend a certain (small) percentage of their available income to obtain these calories (we like to get good "deals"). Since no mega farm or food processing giant has ever gotten rich by selling plain, natural food, they would have to "invent" food-like products that you would actually prefer to plain old natural (and healthy) food. And they would have to make sure you LOVE those foods, to the point of addiction. Judging by the ever expanding waist lines of the general population one would have to conclude that the food industry has been very, very successful in selling *surplus* (inferior) *calories* to us, calories that feed our collective *surplus fat cells*.

"Buy low, sell high." With a little help of the Killer Triple Threat (cheap) ingredients and deft designer-engineering (the "buy/make at a low price" part) on the one hand, and sophisticated marketing and advertising on the other hand (the "sell high" part), we have succeeded in creating a huge industry that has lost sight of its original purpose a long time ago. It's the American Way to search for even more sales and higher profits, and exporting this 'success' story worldwide is the logical next step. The results shouldn't surprise anyone: it is becoming increasingly difficult for formerly smug Germans or French or Japanese or Mexicans to make fun of "fat Americans" since **their** waist lines are expanding rapidly too. They are living proof of the 'success' of the over-processed "Western Diet". "Did you want fries with that?"

WHAT *YOU* CAN DO ABOUT IT

You are out-spent, out-smarted, out-marketed, out-maneuvered every step of the way. Sure, "the government ought to do something about that" – but they aren't. They <u>should</u> subsidize farmers growing a bigger variety of **healthy** vegetables, legumes, root vegetables, fruit, and raising free-range animals without growth hormones. At least, end subsidies for corn and soy, to name just two over-produced agricultural products. They should also enforce existing food safety laws, instead of supporting mega farms growing mono cultures like corn (think cheap HFCS) and soy beans (genetically modified and – via livestock feed – overexposed us to it). It should be a national scandal that $1 buys approximately 100 healthy carrot calories but over 1,000 junk cookie calories, or several hundred calories worth of greasy burgers!

Where is the outrage?
(Or the government for that matter)

Actually, the government is trying. No, really – the obesity crisis is bad for business they have belatedly figured out. So plans are being hatched to tinker with school lunch programs (ketchup no longer a vegetable?), start public awareness campaigns ('effective as always' for youngsters when handed down from daddy-knows-best big government), persuade school vending machine operators to stock healthier choices (even remove sugar-loaded soft drinks altogether – maybe), and revive old-fashioned P.E. classes and classes on nutrition (what, what ... were we thinking of when we cut down on them in the first place???). With all this hoopla and sincere (but naïve) fresh new approach one could be led to believe that the soft drink and junk food manufacturers marketing their unhealthy fare to the next generation are either shaking in their boots, or tearfully returning to the drawing board ("we have sinned, and we are so sorry") and will offer wholesome, healthy food from now on in? HA! As long as there are no laws on the book with "teeth", all we will get in return for all these efforts will be well advertised cosmetic "fixes" to a broken system that will leave their profitable business-as-usual largely the same.

Anyway, I wouldn't hold my breath waiting for the government to get serious anytime soon, if ever. The various food lobbies and processed food industries have a much better donating record than we do. When have YOU - or the asparagus lobby - last donated vast sums of money to a politician's re-election campaign? Do we have a chance? I think we do.

For one, there appears to be an inverse relationship between money spent on food advertising vs. healthfulness of foods. Have you seen the huge advertising campaign for sweet potatoes last year? And the slick infomercials about broccoli ("It's what's for supper")? Neither have I. (Although some avocado growers made a valiant effort some time back and 'honorable mention' has to go to the California raisin commercials.)

However, we DO remember the incessant beat of advertising drums for highly processed, health-claim laden food-like products that were designed to lower our cholesterol, take inches off our waistlines, make us heart-healthy, and provide us with endless energy. The successful results of such advertising are frightening, with the opposite of the claimed benefits often happening. I would go as far as saying that <u>any highly advertised food is probably best avoided</u>. These food-like products are very likely to be over-processed, less healthy than the raw ingredients from which they were derived, and usually chock-a-bloc full of things your body doesn't need or even recognize. There may be the occasional exception, but overall you could do a lot worse than just following this simple, revolutionary advice. You have probably heard the old adage that when you meet a stranger who immediately tells you repeatedly how honest he is, you better hold on to your wallet. Apply this wisdom to highly advertised food 'stuffs' and chances are excellent you will avoid a lot of empty calories.

Therefore the first step on your diet-revolutionary march should be ....

Golden Rule Number 1:
<u>You MUST break the addiction</u> –
and eliminate highly processed foods – and
"Franken-Foods" - from your diet

Easier said than done? Maybe, but "real food" worked for mankind for millions of years. Humans were not hard-wired for refined grains, white sugar, cheap fats or processed foods. As hunter-gatherers, mankind had a more varied, healthier diet of minimally processed or altogether un-processed foods than we enjoy now. And, wide-spread obesity and civilization diseases did not exist. Somewhere during mankind's evolution a few disturbing things happened.

First, we largely discarded a system that was successful for millions of years and replaced it with one that was unproven at best when most humans adopted an agricultural lifestyle making large population centers possible. Later on we compounded this error by refining whole foods for better storage, shipping, handling, and aesthetic reasons. We removed all those nasty ingredients that could spoil real food. Out went the nutritious parts of whole grains, brown rice, and trace elements of (then still scarce) molasses, beet or sugar cane extracts. Equally unfortunate, we started to look at real, whole foods as mere **ingredients** that needed to be "improved", rather than something that could be eaten as is, whole, or cooked or otherwise minimally processed. More and more natural foods had to be "processed", in large part to justify the existence of food processing industries. (In fairness it should be mentioned that the good intent of avoiding food spoilage probably started this trend.) It seems like we lost the ability to look at a simple potato without seeing mashed potatoes or baked potatoes or French fries, all with lots of unnecessary, sometimes unnatural, additional ingredients and cooking methods to "process" them.

Even as recently as 2 or 3 generations ago our grandparents or great-grandparents thrived on simple, minimally processed foods of a wide variety that supplied all the nutrients necessary for health: protein from free-range, grass-fed beef, sheep or even pigs, pasture-roaming chickens and their eggs, wild-caught fish, wholesome legumes, nuts and seeds, organic vegetables and fruit (only they didn't know back then what "organic" was) grown without pesticides, and modest amounts of cooking oils, fats and sweeteners. They ate a bigger variety of foods than we do today (wheat, corn, soy and rice products – all highly processed – make up as much as <u>two thirds</u> of the calories of today's typical American diet). Their food in general tasted better, and they ate only as much as they needed – and they felt no desire to eat any more. Not having ready-to-eat foods available 24/7 surely helped too. They didn't have the "benefit" of government food experts, ever-evolving food pyramids, endless diet books, and food scientists and dieticians, all of which have become necessary "guides" to chaperone you through the jungle of confusing health claims, changing recommendations and the latest pseudo-scientific nutritional breakthroughs.

Things have changed since then – and we can't turn back the clock. Nor should we, having gained so much knowledge about the interaction of food and lifestyles and good health over the last 60-plus years.

Not too many people are in the mood to become hunters and gatherers again. But some things never change: **humans thrive on wholesome, natural, minimally processed foods:**

- Foods that your body can thrive on, not just survive on
- Foods that don't have ingredient lists, or mercifully short ones
- Foods that your great-grandparents would recognize
- Foods that your bodies have adapted to over millions of years
- Foods that don't have mega advertising budgets (call this a Big Red Flag)
- Foods that – and this may come as a surprise to many – taste great just plain, raw or minimally cooked and seasoned.

But you have to break the addiction to over-processed products that pretend to be better than nature's best. That's not an easy task for most people since they never learned to appreciate natural foods unencumbered by added sugars, sodium, cheap fats and a host of chemicals.

Take the lowly baked potato as a prime example. Judging by the perplexed look I get whenever I order a plain baked potato with nothing on or in it, I am willing to bet that most people wouldn't know what to do with a potato that wasn't loaded with butter, sour cream, cheese, chives, (fatty) chopped meat, sauces and possibly other toppings. Voilà – the healthy, unprocessed, low-cal but highly nutritional potato has been degraded to a <u>delivery system</u> for some of the unhealthiest things known to mankind. All a really good baked potato needs (and you probably won't find a good potato at your local supermarket) is a little salt sprinkled on top, possibly a little extra virgin olive oil, and lo and behold, you can actually taste the potato. So skip the unhealthy toppings and eat that crunchy, fiber-rich skin, provided it's an organic potato that has been thoroughly cleaned. Same story with the even-healthier sweet potato – it doesn't need to float in maple syrup nor does it have to be covered with boatloads of sugary marshmallows, butter (or worse, non-dairy "spread") or anything else. Just a knife and a fork, possibly a little salt, and a small amount of sweetener if you must. Try it sometime – you might get a pleasant surprise.

Apply this concept to all foods you put on your plate: steamed broccoli without au gratin cheese; a crisp apple instead of apple pie; a tossed garden salad with a little vinaigrette, not iceberg lettuce and a token (tasteless) tomato drowned in ranch dressing; plain or slightly salted nuts instead of pecan pie; steamed fresh fish in a light ginger or soy broth vs. that same fish battered and deep-fried. Enjoy **real** peanut butter vs. peanut butter with hydrogenated fats, sugars, palm oil, preservatives, stabilizers, etc. Stir up a jar of Laura Scudder's All Natural Old-Fashioned Peanut Butter® (hints: store jar upside down for a few days prior to stirring; and a hand-mixer is a handy gadget to have), take one taste, and you'll never go back to "Skip-It" brands.

"Plain" or "minimally processed" doesn't mean without seasoning and devoid of taste. Au contraire: avail yourself of fresh herbs, sea salt, freshly ground pepper and other spices to bring out the flavors and add healthful ingredients. Still not convinced?   Find a *real Oriental* restaurant or supermarket near you ("American-Chinese" doesn't count, especially if an all-you-can-eat buffet is involved) and discover a whole world of Chinese, Indian, Thai, Vietnamese, Korean, and Malaysian spices, and you will never again have a boring meal of bland chicken breast, iceberg lettuce and French fries. Remember – advertising works or corporations wouldn't spend billions of dollars on it. Don't fall for it – don't have your food choices dictated by slick advertising. The health-iest foods are rarely, if ever advertised, and offer the best nutritional return on your food dollar investment.

Still not convinced you can live without your favorite over-processed food? Consider this: the foods you like the most are *probably* deeply rooted in your childhood experiences and are *definitely* the ones you eat the most. That's right, if you eat a lot of cheese (or chocolate, or greasy burgers, or you-name-it) you become mildly addicted to it and want to eat more and more of it. This is bad news – but you can turn it to your advantage by starting to eat healthy, unprocessed foods more often (surely you can think of one or two you like …). You will notice that the ho-hum organic red pepper or a plain roasted sweet potato (just to name two examples) can grow on you to the point where you want to eat some every day. Now that would be a *good* food addiction (assuming you don't go overboard on any single food, at the expense of a balanced diet).

A word about **"Franken-Foods"**: for one, it's not obvious that they are, or else we would never buy them. For example, shouldn't some delicious, un-processed turkey meat be near the top of your shopping list? Not if the poor birds have been raised on an unnatural fast weight-gain food-like cocktail of cheap ingredients (many of them grown in depleted soils), antibiotics, growth hormones, and enough chemicals to have a significant negative health impact. Add animal cruelty that would be considered punishable abuse if we treated pets that way, unsanitary conditions (combated by powerful chemicals), and a near-complete lack of government inspections, and you may want to re-think that Thanksgiving Special gobbler, which, by-the-way, can't even walk anymore (much less reproduce). And things are equally bad and sometimes worse, for commercially-raised chickens and their eggs, most farm-raised fish and seafood, veal (the poster child for animal cruelty), beef, pigs, and most of the animal by-products where we apply the "head in the sand" mentality – think hot dogs, hamburgers and a huge array of similarly processed foods, as well as pesticide-laden produce grown on mega farms in depleted soils.

What can <u>you</u> do about it? Recognize these "Franken-Foods" and just say **no!**

Golden Rule Number 2: <u>Have 5-6 small meals a day</u>

Sure, Moms worldwide were right when they dispensed conventional wisdom like "3 square meals a day" and "eat your vegetables", and their track record speaks for itself. The obesity crisis didn't start until mothers as dietary 'goddesses' were replaced first by government 'experts', then by scientists and advertising executives of giant food processors. But we can do even better than "Mom" did back then, with the added knowledge of proven research, and – to no small extent – trial and error as to what worked and what didn't. Staying with the Golden Rule Number Two, we have to tweak Mom's advice only slightly: "3 small meals and 2-3 healthy, small snacks a day", consisting of mostly unprocessed foods, and <u>each meal or snack balanced with the right amounts of protein, carbohydrates, and fat</u>. Two extra meals of course is not a free pass to extra calories: each meal or snack should be in the 200 – 600 (max.!) calorie range, depending on a variety of factors such as age, sex, physical activity level, weight, height, etc. You may want to think long and hard about the 300-400 calories of chips and dips, or white bread and butter you consume before the actual meal arrives. Or adding that 700-calorie slice of death-by-chocolate cake to your steak dinner - "à la mode" of course.

IMPORTANT: "grazing" all day is not the answer! You must give the stomach time to process each meal and move it down the digestive tract before feeding it again! It is these "gaps" between meals during which you don't ingest anything (except water, or calorie-free beverages) that are the 'secret ingredient' in your successful weight loss strategy. This is not to be confused with fasting, or starving yourself; when the time is right (you feel hungry) by all means feed your body, even if that means moving up a meal or a snack, or having an additional snack. Call it *3 balanced meals, 2 balanced snacks, and <u>4 periods in-between of letting the stomach do its work uninterrupted.</u>*

So how do you know if a given meal is big enough to sustain you until the next snack? Well, you could count calories. Estimate your daily requirements by starting with your BMR (basal metabolic rate – the number of calories you need just to "keep the lights on"), then add caloric expenditures for various daily activities (surf the web, or have a professional do it for you – either way you end up with guestimates at best), divide by the number of meals and snacks you plan to have, and you get a pretty good idea how much to eat at any given time. This can be a great exercise, but it's tedious, and fraught with pitfalls, like having to rely on the accuracy of food labels (they aren't), interpreting what a "medium banana" or a "small orange" is, and having to measure or weigh every single ingredient of your meal. This can be depressing – literally! Even then, standard calorie charts vary wildly and the cumulative margins of error will result in little more than WEGs – wild, educated guesses. Dining out? Good luck getting some nutritional data at all, much less *accurate* data (calories and fat are typically under-reported). <u>You'll never last.</u>

You are much better off trusting your instincts – assuming you have given your body and brain a chance by eliminating foods that overload and misguide your sensory receptors. You know how they say that "you never forget how to ride a bike"? It's true of course. Even if you haven't ridden a bike in 30 years, if you swing your leg over one and start to pedal, you'll take off - albeit with a little wobble at first. Same with food portions: when kids can choose their own portion sizes rather than having somebody else fill their plate (most likely to overflow), they usually pick just the right amount they need – and then stop. Sometimes it's a big, heaping plate, sometimes a tiny snack. And you still have that same, if under-used, skill. You can prepare one meal at a time, put all the ingredients on a plate or in a bowl, look at it, and instinctively feel that yes, this meal will tide me over until the next meal or snack, 3-4 short hours later. Or no, this is way too much (put part of it away for another meal). Practice, and after a few <u>trial and error</u> sessions (think of the "wobble" part of that first bicycle ride after many years), chances are you'll get the portion sizes right. And remember: no second servings! It is generally accepted that it takes approximately 25 minutes for the brain to receive the "sated" signal from the stomach (certainly a design flaw in the human species), so **don't even think about seconds and walk away** from the dinner table and the refrigerator. Put a timing device to good use, and consider all food off-limits until the time is up – at which point you should not be the least bit hungry anymore. If you truly erred on the low side of calories you can have your next snack a little bit earlier, or have a slightly larger meal next time. <u>You should feel good and (slightly) hungry for every meal, but not to the point of being ravenous.</u> If you are not you can either delay the meal, or even cancel it. **Sometimes the best meal to have is ... no meal at all!**

Micro-managing your daily meal only *sounds* tedious or time consuming, but having a <u>plan</u> will insure that you don't lose track of your overall goal of either losing or maintaining weight. Oh, and did you know that Americans watch an average of THREE to FIVE hours of television every day? (Where do they find the time???). I just mention this to put a wooden stake through the heart of the "I don't have the time to plan my meals" argument. You have to decide what's more important to you – feeling great, being healthy, and enjoying quality of life in general, or the latest episode of "American Idol". Think about that for a moment.

Golden Rule Number 3:
Don't worry about that *perfect* ratio of carbs, protein and fat

Is there a perfect ratio? Yes – several of them actually. Just ask 10 people (scientists, dieticians, athletic coaches, government experts, etc.) and chances are you'll get 10 different "perfect" answers. "1-2-3" is the way to go, some say (1 part fat, 2 parts protein, and 3 parts carbs). No, the ratio we should all aim for is 65% carbs, 20% protein, and 15% fats. Or was that 60-25-15? Or 70-20-10? Or 60-20-20? Some athletes maintain that the 40-30-30 diet brings best results – 40% carbs, 30% protein, and 30% fats. And on and on the debate continues, changing every season. Even if that mythical "perfect" ratio was once and for all determined, for whom would it be perfect? – the teenage track team member or her 70-year old grandmother? The 45-year old couch potato or the 60-year old marathon veteran? The overweight heart-attack-victim waiting to happen or the 110 lbs. fashion model training for her first triathlon? Certainly it can't be the same for all, all the time. More importantly, how much time and effort and education do you need to hit that perfect ratio, day-in, day-out? We are back to counting calories, one by one - how much fun would that be, and how long would you last? And who has all the detailed information on every single thing you eat every day, since many of the healthiest things aren't even labeled (vegetables, fruit), some of the not so healthy ones (think fast-food and other restaurants) may not be available, and the nutritional data that is available varies depending on which book or website you choose? Unless you have a team of nutrition experts weigh and evaluate every single calorie before you eat anything you'll never come even close to being on target for your "perfect" ratio of nutrients.

There's got to be a better way, and there is: make sure that the calories in your meal come approximately ½ **to 2/3 from carbohydrates** (vegetables, fruit, legumes, root vegetables), and the rest from **quality proteins**. Think 3-4oz of protein – not a "trim cut 8oz" monster (or more!) for one meal. Fats quite often take care of themselves since they are part of so many foods (animal proteins, tofu, nuts, seeds, legumes, avocado, etc.), but if any particular meal does not contain fat already, or has not been prepared with healthy oils or fat add some fat in the form of nuts or seeds. There are other foods that should be included with some meals, and we'll address them later, but the above snap shot represents the basic composition. That's it. It's that easy - no need to worry about getting too much or too little of one food group vs. the other. Chances are it will all even out at your next meal if you follow the simple guidelines above. Just make sure that each and every meal is balanced, and contains some protein, some complex carbs, and some healthy fats. And not every meal must or should include animal proteins. Any combination of legumes and nuts, or legumes and seeds, or legumes and whole grains will result in a quality protein containing all essential amino acids, as will tofu and tempeh.

Golden Rule Number 4: don't fall into the "exclusionary diet" trap

Trying to avoid all foods or food-like products that are associated with a little bad-for-you baggage can soon leave you trying to exist on nuts that fell off the pecan tree in your backyard and vegetables that died a natural death (after a long, happy life). Not very balanced or healthy. Don't go there. Sometimes choosing the lesser of the 2 (or more) evils will get you through the day better than the "holier than the pope" approach to food. "Compromise" need not be a four-letter word. Life isn't perfect – read up in the chapter of "Good vs. Bad Foods" for more info.

Golden Rule Number 5: To be truly healthy you must stay physically active

The good news is we are not talking about training for a marathon here! <u>You are doing a lot of exercising already</u>, without even realizing it and being fit enough to be able to run a marathon at any given moment is not required (but it wouldn't hurt). Getting out of bed, moving around the house, doing chores, driving to work, picking up things, playing with children, shopping, etc. all have the effect of keeping our muscles active by exercising them. Without doing any of this we would be confined to bed in a very short period of time, helpless and sick. In some instances, these everyday actions and chores are all the body needs. Think of many cultures in Europe, Asia, or S. America, where people still <u>walk</u> a lot instead of driving, still spend many hours attending to their gardens, still take stairs instead of using elevators or escalators, still use bicycles for daily transportation or for weekend getaways, or still have a physically active job. So yes, if you have a very active lifestyle, and limit your caloric intake, you probably can attain **"health status"** without additional structured exercise.

But … this kind of lifestyle is not typical for Americans: we drive everywhere, park as close to the entrance as possible (like, at the gym), avoid climbing stairs whenever possible, and use drive-thru lanes - to pick up our donuts, among other things! Human beings need more activity than that, especially once life becomes more sedentary and settled somewhere north of 40 or so years. Before that, youthful metabolism, more spontaneous activities, and general lack of health issues combine to lull us into a sense of security that we don't really need to exercise beyond a game of touch football on 4th of July. It doesn't help that as a society we have made "exercise" synonymous with pain, sweat, discomfort, and quite often punishment (think of that extra lap you had to run on the high school track if your behavior was deemed inappropriate), while sweets, cookies, ice cream, and dessert were given out as "rewards" for good behavior, having met a goal, or acing a test. This cultural "baggage" that burdens exercise is hard to overcome for many, but we know that a healthy lifestyle without meaningful time spent on physical activity is a myth perpetrated by the high priests of quick-fix diets, junk weight loss plans and miracle weight loss pills.

So can you lead a healthy life without exercising?

Before I answer that question, let me ask you this: why would you want to exclude exercising? You'd deprive yourself of a powerful "one-two" punch in your battle of the bulge. If you had to step into a boxing ring to fight a big, strong opponent (surplus calories – the heavy weight champion), would you fight him with one arm tied behind your back? I hope not! Sure, a strict diet alone might take the weight off, but it would be a much harder, longer, and potentially unhealthier battle. And you are more likely to take the weight off in the first place and then keep it off if you incorporate a meaningful, regular physical activity program. Most important, exercising / physical activity just plain makes us feel good! No 'delayed benefits' here that you won't reap until you are 90 (that will come as a bonus), but feel-good rewards right then and there, after you are done, and for the rest of the day.

Maybe it's best to refer to "physical activity" rather than structured exercising. Are you one of those people that just can't sit still? Excellent! Assuming your job allows it, and you don't stay idle for long outside of your job, this will be your best defense against some illnesses associated with a sedentary lifestyle. Sitting for long periods at a time has now been shown to be a separate risk factor for cardiovascular disease, independent of other activities. Therefore you can't "make up" for excessive sitting with rigorous after-hours or weekend warrior-type workouts, including serious athletic endeavors. They will not undo the damage you incur sitting your life away. Never mind the term "couch potato". Being a "chair knödel" is potentially much more dangerous. This would possibly explain how some seemingly fit and active people can keel over from a heart attack without warning. So don't just sit there – do something, get out of that chair, for a healthier heart, posture, back, hips, spine, shoulders, etc.

But back to the original question as to whether it is possible to get / remain healthy without exercising. By that I mean maintaining a weight that keeps you below the "overweight" category and protects you from civilization's many diseases. **Maybe**, but you are making it a lot harder for yourself, and will fall short of true "quality of life". Even then you would have to emulate the lifestyle of people of other, more active cultures, as outlined above, and adopt healthy eating habits, which this book will show you. Never mind the "Mediterranean Diet" – call it the *Mediterranean Lifestyle* (such as we think it was in the 50-ies and 60-ies): reduce the time you spend in front of the TV or the computer from hours to minutes. As time spent sitting in front of these appliances has increased, our overall activity levels have decreased, or rather *plummeted*. Walk instead of drive whenever possible. Discover stairs and avoid elevators, when practical. Don't spend 10 minutes curving around parking lots to get that spot closest to the entrance, but deliberately park away from the entrance and walk (bonus: you may find a shady parking spot, and nobody will slam his shopping cart into your car). Commute on foot or by bicycle, if you can safely do so. Sit on a stability ball instead of comfy armchair (I bet you didn't know these were all the rage in Greece in the 50-ies!). Feed off the endless energy of kids by playing outdoors with them, instead of watching a movie with them. Let the dog (or the cat) have the couch and work on your garden (or shovel snow) instead. Better yet, take that dog out for a long walk. And walk to the cubicle down the hall to talk to your co-worker, instead of sending an e-mail. Make it your very own "competition" to see what stationery habits in your life you can replace with active, moving activities. All these "negligible" extra calories burned can add up to 200 or more calories a day – up to 800 calories if you do serious manual chores. That's over 70.000 calories (at a minimum) in a year, or the equivalent of losing (or gaining) 20 lbs. or more, assuming you don't "make up for it" at the dinner table. And with incremental extra calories burned throughout the day, you will be less tempted to "reward" yourself – with food of course – like you might do after burning the same amount with one sweat-inducing workout session.

Still, my conviction is that **anybody over 40 cannot maintain a healthy weight and become or remain truly fit and healthy**

without regular exercise consisting of both cardio and resistance workouts. Are there exceptions to the rule – are there people who are slim but don't ever work up a sweat? Maybe – but how many of them are malnourished, like the aging diva who starves herself, but can still squeeze her body into the same size jeans she wore 30 years ago? And of course this need to get active doesn't exactly start the day after your 40th birthday: being physically active beyond daily routines should start well before then (it should really never stop after structured school-based sports are no longer part of your life). But somewhere in your life before mid-life crisis sets in you may want to give some thought to picking up an activity you enjoy instead of buying a Harley or a Corvette. Sure, one can survive without ever breaking a sweat, but remember, _all those who cannot find time for health will have to find time for disease,_ many of which are preventable. They will also age before their time, lose muscle mass (and functional strength with it) at a rapid pace, and generally lose quality - and quantity – of life.

The good news: it doesn't take as much time and effort as many non-exercisers believe to go to the next level – the **"fit status"**. No ex-Olympian needed to coach you into shape, or boot camps to survive. A little goes a long way, as long as you make exercise a regular part of your life. Like Gus does, for example. Gus is a healthy-looking gentleman in the weight room of the Y where I work out. He is 85 years old, slim, active, enjoys his short workouts and the camaraderie of like-minded people around him. He looks and acts like he is a decade younger – and a long way from searching for an assisted-living center. And then there is Beth, a young chick in comparison in the same Y. She is a fitness instructor, and looks trim and fit enough that you think she's ready to run the Boston marathon on an hour's notice. Not bad for an 80-year old! See the chapter "An Active Lifestyle" for the information that could improve your life dramatically, but here's a quick primer of what you can – and should – do to keep in shape:

- 30-60 minutes of uninterrupted cardio workouts, 3-5 times per week. Sure, a brisk run or a few thousand yards of swimming will do the trick, but so will vigorous walks, or any other number of "user-friendly" activities that appeal to you. And some of that time has to be spent in a high intensity mode for best results (definitely check with your doctor before starting a new, vigorous workout schedule!). The good news: if you include short bursts of high intensity you can save yourself as much as half your steady-state boring time spent on your favorite activity (although you should probably not exercise less than 30 minutes per cardio session). Wouldn't 30 minutes of cardio interspersed with a few hard efforts lasting 1-5 minutes be preferable to slogging one hour watching mind-numbing TV shows? Your workout will be more effective, shorter, and will have more of an impact on overall health and weight reduction.

- 2-3 sessions in the weight room per week, or at-home workouts engaging in resistance-bearing exercises. Get professional advice on a well rounded program. No, you won't bulk up – unless you plan to do some heavy lifting for several hours during 6 days of the week and you have Schwarzenegger-like genes and/or "do" steroids.

- 2-3 workouts specifically targeting core strength and stretching. Again, get your bearings from a health care professional or personal trainer at your local gym, and get an introductory course on types of exercises, and good form. No need to schedule 2-3 additional workouts, but rather add these core & stretch routines to your weight room exercises. Separate Yoga or Pilates sessions would also be good options.

- Like any new physical activity, check with your doctor before embarking on any new and/or strenuous workout regime. Don't risk your health in the quest of improving it. And don't race yourself in shape. Having been inactive for years and carrying some extra weight because of it, does not qualify you for the accelerated 6-week (or even 6 month) marathon training program. What's safe for everybody is **not** sitting around too long at any given time, and water-based workouts are suitable for all but the most serious medical cases.

- Don't expect results overnight – or even in a week or two. But, after 6 or more weeks you will! Yes, that means a lot of sweat equity with little to show in return at first. The answer is not to throw your arms up ("it's just not working for me") but to <u>persevere.</u> It takes approx. 6 weeks of regular exercise for results to be noticeable, <u>become ingrained</u> as a habit, and for physiological and biomechanical changes to be profound. Take-home lesson: plan for it, get active <u>now</u>, and don't quit. You <u>will</u> notice positive changes.
- Probably the best way to gain health benefits from physical activity is to get **athletic**! Once your weight is under control and you have been working out on a regular basis, go ahead and enter that 5K! Just making that commitment can be a powerful motivator to 'do the right things' and before you know it maintaining a healthy weight will be a side benefit of your quest to improve in your chosen athletic field. Running is not your thing? Sign up for an organized bike ride, or Pilate's class, tennis lessons, or masters swimming – even shuffle board in your later years: surely there is a healthy activity that you'll enjoy doing, alone or as part of a group.

Still, getting "healthy" or "fit" or "athletic" will not solve all of life's problems. Sorry. However, you will be able to <u>cope better</u> with stress, frustrations, and anxiety, thereby "shrinking" the problems – and that's scientifically proven. Wouldn't that be good enough to settle for? Give it a try for 6 weeks or more and see for yourself. How to get started? Cut out one hour of TV time in the evening, get up an hour earlier to exercise, and dedicate that hour to your health - see the chapter "An active lifestyle" for help. Can't possibly get out of bed that early? If you had to catch a plane you could. If you had to drive all day to a family reunion you could. If you wanted to catch the early-bird special Thanks-giving Sale you could. It can't be <u>that</u> hard then. And if your life may depend on it you should be able to also.

<u>Tomorrow morning would be a great time to start!</u>

IT'S NOT [only] *WHAT* YOU EAT – IT'S *WHEN* YOU EAT IT

And **"how much you eat at any given meal"** too. Oh, and **"how often you eat"**.

Sound complicated? It doesn't have to be, so let's revisit and expand **Golden Rule Number 2**:

3 balanced meals a day / 2 snack-sized meals a day (mid-morning / mid-afternoon) / 200-600 cal. each (and NO grazing in between!)

Keep in mind that the total amount of ingested calories does NOT go up just because the number of "feedings" goes up! Some meals will have to be "downsized". And 600 cal. is on the high side – preferably those main meals will be a little bit smaller and less filling.

1. Three balanced meals: yup, just like Mom told you. "Balanced" means that half or more of your plate (aim for 2/3) should be covered by raw or minimally processed vegetables, or root vegetables, or fresh fruit. The next largest section on your plate should have a quality source of protein on it (25-35%). If there is no fat on your plate (no avocados, no fatty meats, no nuts, seeds, legumes, or your food has not been prepared with fat) add some nuts or seeds, or add one of the healthy oils. For details as to what kinds of proteins, fats, and oils to include, refer to the chapter on "BASICS".

2. 2 snack-sized meals: these are optional – don't force yourself to eat them if you are not hungry because you had a bigger breakfast or lunch than you should have. Skipping these snacks is a good way to "catch" yourself if you have overeaten. Assuming you judged breakfast and lunch portion sizes right, chances are you will feel hungry by mid-morning and again by mid-afternoon. That's when you come prepared and don't fall prey to the snack vending machine, which has inferior choices at higher prices. And just because this "mini-meal" is referred to as a snack, it is not a license for junk food. It can still be balanced: an apple with a small handful of a nut-legume mix (peanuts – legumes, and "real" nuts) would be a good example. Or a small serving of oatmeal (100 cal

46

      pouch) with a few peanuts, raisins, ground flax seeds, and a banana. Or a small soy yoghurt with blueberries. Use your imagination and keep it small, simple, and easy to prepare and bring with you.

3.   200-600 calories: why such relatively small portions? For one because you are adding 2 "mini-meals" to the 3 "regular" meals you consume already (hopefully). Plus, the goal is to practice the "just-in-time" inventory system, where no excess calories will be stored in that ungainly storage area for future uses – the fat warehouse.

As for "*what*" to eat, refer to the "BASICS" chapter for recommended healthy choices. How about portion sizes? As mentioned in the chapter "EATING MORE IS NOT THE ANSWER", Golden Rule No. 2. And while we are on the subject of having more than just the 3 traditional meals: maybe you have heard this before, or – I hope not – have practiced this approach yourself, which is still "out there". "I want to lose weight, so I will only have one meal a day" (usually delivered with the smug demeanor of a martyr). That happens to be the perfect recipe for **gaining** weight! Why? Our ancestral survival instincts kick in. The body is led to believe that no food will be forthcoming for a while and goes into starvation-survival mode (after that one, huge meal), desperately holding on to those calories and slowing down your metabolism. If some people somehow manage to keep their weight in a healthy range using this "system", more likely than not they'll develop nutritional deficiencies. Don't take your body down that road. Instead, keep it happily out of starvation mode with several small meals throughout the day, metabolism all revved up.

THE BASICS

You don't have to be a mechanical engineer or a computer wizard to drive a car. You can be a pretty good driver just by knowing certain basics. Like the fact that the car has an engine, that the engine needs quality fuel to perform, tires have to be inflated within a certain pressure range, and oil has to be changed every so often. You know there is a magical electrical system that's required for more than just the vanity lights, hydraulics that make your life easier steering and braking, and you know that a little maintenance will go a long way to keep you from being stranded in the middle of nowhere.

The same concept applies to nutritional and lifestyle factors. You don't need to have a Master's degree in nutrition, but you should know some basic information about how your body works and what it needs. After all, you want it to work smoothly, without breakdowns or tows to the service station, especially since the body's service stations are hospitals. (And you thought car repairs were expensive.) So yes, it helps to know the basics.

First, some bad news: as far as the human body is concerned you don't get to choose the model, like you would with a car. You are born with the body that you have. You can't pick a Michael Phelps or a Jackie Joyner-Kersee model. No upgrades, exchanges or trade-ins, sorry. And since you only have that one model for your whole life it might be a good idea to take good care of it – wouldn't you baby your car if you knew it would have to last you a lifetime? And don't bemoan the fact that you got stuck with a gas guzzler ("body") instead of a super-efficient model. That hybrid that's advertised as getting 40 mpg will be hard-pressed to get 30 mpg if its owner has a lead foot. Yet I can get a real-world 35 mpg on the highway with a minivan that's advertised as only getting 26 mpg on open roads. And chances are you'll drive your Chevette long after the same year model Jaguar is filling up a landfill if you treated your Chevette with a lot of TLC vs. having abused the Jag. It's all about what you make with what you've got.

To start with, here's a good basic rule: *don't put premium gasoline into your gas tank, and junk food into your body.* Self-explanatory you say? One would think so, yet it doesn't explain all the Lexuses, BMWs and Mercs lining up in the donut store drive-through lane. Think about that for a minute. You probably know already what all falls into the junk food category (although there may be some healthy-appearing surprises in there), but when it comes to premium fuel for your body it can get complicated. For one, there is no consensus as to what constitutes the "perfect" diet; probably there are several very good, if not "perfect" ways to fuel your body.

Let's look at **what is absolutely required for humans to survive – and thrive**: Forget about 4, 5 or even 6 major food groups, and let's break it down into the basic building blocks – there are just three:

- Protein
- Carbohydrates
- Oils & Fats

Of course there are also other, all-important ingredients necessary for life: clean air, clean water, and physical activity, as well as herbs, spices, fiber - all of which can increase the quality of life.

- **Protein:** no doubt about it – you cannot survive long without it. Protein is required for growth, cell repair, recovery, enzyme production, regulation of hormones, fighting off disease, etc., and even as a source of energy (although it takes a back seat to carbohydrates there). It would stand to reason that since "you are what you eat", quality is the most important criteria when choosing protein sources, assuming sufficient **quantity** of protein is consumed. How much is enough: opinions vary, and "one size does not fit all", but **25-35%** of your total caloric intake should work for most people. Endurance athletes or weightlifters in general have higher requirements than sedentary adults, as do growing children, people recovering from injuries or disease and other, special populations. More on that later.

• **Carbohydrates:** pure muscle fuel – how can anybody try to sell you an "all protein / no carb" junk-science diet? Obviously only somebody who never tried it before for any length of time; it's not a pretty picture. It's horrible. You 'bonk', feel and look like the walking wounded (or dead), performance goals give way to just 'making it', and your movements become uncoordinated – truly a danger to yourself and others. Don't go there. Quality carbohydrate-rich foods are high-octane fuel for your body, and the best source of energy for daily human functions and athletic performance are *complex carbohydrates*.

Where do you find them? Mostly in legumes, root vegetables, vegetables, fruit, and whole grains. Avoid high intake of <u>simple carbohydrates</u> found in plain sugar and syrups, but also in natural sweeteners such as honey, maple syrup, molasses, and to some extent in fruit. How much is enough? Conventional wisdom considers 65% to be the magic number, but nutritional C.W. has not always served us too well, and **40-50%** of total calories coming from mostly complex carbohydrates should fuel the average human quite nicely, without crowding out healthy proteins and fats. Strenuous manual labor or preparing for athletic endurance events (as well as during and right afterwards) would require a somewhat higher intake – as much as 65% or more.

• **Fats and Oils:** despite some of them justly being referred to as "essential" fats, they were the bogeymen of 'advanced' food scientists of the 70-ies and 80-ies – and some unenlightened die-hards of the 21st century. "Low-fat" trumped the common sense of a tried-and-proven human food component, and "no-fat" soon trumped "low fat". "9 evil calories of fat" vs. "only 4 calories of saintly carbohydrates" per gram – it seemed like such a slam dunk. Everybody did the math, many dutifully changed their eating habits – and the obesity crises began in earnest. When America awoke from this carb-induced obesity hangover a few years later the damage was done. Oh, and the number of heart attacks did <u>not</u> go down either, as eagerly claimed by pro low-fat diet advocates. Rather, the better <u>survival rates</u> of same (compliments of medical advances) gave at least the *appearance* of success, so at first it was easy to "declare victory and leave". Suffice it to say, that yes, oils and fats, either as a natural part of food (nuts, seeds, vegetables, meat, eggs, fish, etc.) or as an added ingredient in the form of healthy oils and fats, were, are, and always will be part of a healthy diet.

What is worrisome however is where most Americans get their fat – a whopping 60% from animal sources! Think cholesterol & saturated fats, not to mention quality concerns, and then re-think your dietary habits. How much fat is really enough? It depends on your age, weight, activity level, cultural background, and many other factors, but I don't think reducing total fat consumption below 15% is a healthy proposition. Many healthy population groups consume as much as 50% of (healthy) fats and thrive. As a general rule you should aim to consume **20-30%** of your calories in the form of healthy fats. (Keep in mind that one innocent-looking tablespoon of any oil typically packs 120 calories!). Even skinny endurance runners who fell into the trap of ultra-low fat diets noticed performance improvements once moderate amounts of fat were added back into their diets. Monounsaturated, polyunsaturated, and small amounts of saturated fats all have a place in a healthy diet – but transfats and fully hydrogenated or partially hydrogenated fats **do not** (except for small amounts of

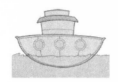 natural transfats from animal sources). Review the best fats to include in your diet below, in the section "SAFE AND HEALTHY FOODS WITHIN THE VARIOUS FOOD GROUPS OF THE FOOD ARK™".

Also, no discussion on dietary fat intake should miss mentioning one particularly worrisome development in reference *to the make-up of fats* in mankind's diet. While early humans' diets probably had a ratio of 1:1 to 1:4 of omega-3 to omega-6 fatty acids, that healthy profile has deteriorated to an unhealthy 1:20! Thank the inclusion of dairy products, grains, highly processed oils, carbohydrates, today's domesticated meats (vs. wild game and wild-caught fish), and alcohol for that significant negative impact on human health. Research indicates that the excess omega-6 f.a. consumption in much of the Western world is partly to blame for many diseases, particularly the so-called "lifestyle diseases" that could be reduced tremendously if appropriate lifestyle changes would be adopted. Think cardiovascular disease, diabetes, obesity, hypertension, many types of cancer and inflammatory diseases, such as rheumatoid arthritis.

- Not necessarily a food, but more important for survival, is **water**. Humans can survive for a week or longer without food, but will only last 2-3 days without water. However, ingest polluted water, or water unfit for human consumption (salt water), and life-sustaining water will do just the opposite – extinguish life in a short period of time. What's the gold standard? Look no further than good old cheap tap water (in most, but not all communities in industrialized countries) – as long as it has been filtered, preferably by a 5-step reverse osmosis filtering process. Such filtration devices are readily available for under $300.00 and are easily installed under the kitchen sink. Once installed there are no expensive plastic bottles to buy (avoiding an environmental nightmare) or worry about leached chemicals. Over the life of these R.O. systems the cost of clean water is reduced to pennies a gallon, so you won't feel bad using this water to cook with, steam vegetables, and prepare teas or coffees. It's an investment in your health that will pay for itself within a year or two, compared to buying bottled water. And while you are at it, use glass bottles whenever possible to avoid compounds from plastic containers leaching into your drinking water and to avoid adding to your local landfill.

- What about **fiber**? Ideally, if you choose only natural, minimally processed, 'real' foods of a wide variety and in the right proportions, you should get all the fiber your body needs to thrive - keeping in mind that dietary fiber is only found in plant foods. Consequently your best insurance policy for a healthy diet that meets all your nutritional requirements in general, and fiber requirements in particular, is, and always will be, a diet high in vegetables and fruits (organic if possible), root vegetables, quality proteins, nuts, and seeds, supplemented by "good fats" if dietary fat intake is low. If additional fiber is needed, increasing the amount of fresh, raw vegetables, fruit, and dried fruit will raise fiber intake naturally. Unless there are medical conditions that warrant such (check with your doctor first), commercial laxatives should be avoided at all costs! Both artificial and herb-based laxatives are not natural for your body, possibly contain harmful ingredients, and quite often lead to a dependency on them, reducing the efficiency of the body's natural digestive & elimination processes. Potentially hazardous side affects can also include potassium depletion and liver damage.

"Just say no" - <u>there is a better way</u> to "stay regular", if all else fails. Yes, there is a natural food – in combination with a healthy, fiber-rich diet and generous amounts of liquids - that is better than any other at providing healthy, nutritious, and non-addictive fiber, with all the benefits and none of the drawbacks. It even tastes good and adds healthy omega-3 fatty acids to your diet. Does this sound like a miracle food? Well it is, in a way, and it is **(organic) ground flaxseed meal.** And no, eating a grease-trap muffin sprinkled with a few whole flax seeds will not do anything for you, except deliver unhealthy surplus calories.

The human stomach cannot break down the tough outer shell of flax seeds in their natural state, and only after grinding them will they be useful for you. It's best to buy flax seeds whole and grind them at home in a coffee grinder (when your coffee-loving spouse isn't around), or buy freshly ground flaxseed meal in the supermarket. Either version should be kept in the freezer (don't worry, it will not clump/freeze together) since the oil in flax seeds becomes rancid quickly after exposure to air. How much is enough? 1-3 tablespoons will do, although you may start out with less than that. *More is not better!* How to include it in your diet? I find that the best way to make sure you consume enough is by setting out 1-3 table spoons in a suitable container every day, and making sure you consume it all by the end of the day, then set out another batch for the next day. Mix it into fruit juices, teas, salads, cereals, dips & sauces, peanut butter, casseroles, or any other food you can think of. It adds a nice nutty flavor, and tends to thicken up liquids or sauces. Remember: talking about being "regular" is only marginally funny until you are not regular anymore. That's when it can become a serious health hazard, way beyond a little discomfort. Constipation will eventually lead to what is best described as 'internal self-poisoning' that will affect every organ and every cell in your body. No laughing matter.

FOOD PYRAMIDS

I don't know about you, but I have lost track of – and interest in – how many different food pyramids are out there at this time, with new ones arriving every day it seems. There are probably more of them than there were pyramids in all of ancient Egypt!

They all have similar basic flaws:

- Usually there is no differentiation between refined and whole grains. This flaw is monumental - the government experts failed us on that one. *Refined grains should be the broad foundation of another pyramid – the civilization disease pyramid!* Think cancers, high blood pressure, adult-onset diabetes, obesity and all the complications associated with it. Mankind survived for millions of years quite nicely without agriculture in general and grains in particular - and presumably also without any of the above diseases. Since mankind hasn't fared so well in the last 10,000-some years since the wide-spread adoption of grains, even their inclusion in food pyramids should be open to debate. At the very least grains should have been specified as "whole grains only", although one cannot help but wonder if pur-veyors of refined grain products "influenced" their gener-alized inclusion and pushed the differentiation between whole and processed grains into nutritional oblivion. Cer-tainly the prominence of that food group would suggest such: 11 slices of plain white accordion bread would have met the "grain" requirements for a day!

- Milk and dairy products have their own huge piece of the (pyramid) pie? Based on *what* evidence? The fact that the colostrum of an altogether different species was elevated to a critical part of the food pyramid is more indicative of how powerful the dairy lobby is, than it is of the actual importance and *healthfulness* of dairy products. Early humans were genetically "wired" to reject milk of any kind beyond nursing time, - and would get sick consuming it.

In many cultures around the world the consumption of milk for adults is considered unusual or downright repulsive. When some Europeans' genetic predisposition to reject milk was "turned off" in relatively recent history (5000 years, give or take), it gave them access to a new protein that helped them survive under tough conditions. Just because this "survival adaptation" occurred doesn't necessarily make a food "healthy" or desirable for all humans, as witnessed by widespread lactose intolerance in many population groups. Selling drugs to Native Americans, Blacks, and Hispanics – when majorities of all these population groups are lactose intolerant (as are a growing number of European-Americans) - so they can "tolerate" a food their body naturally rejects appears to be a cynical profit-driven strategy, and does not constitute responsible health management. It is time to re-think our relationship with dairy and wipe the milk moustaches from grown-ups' faces.

- Meats, seafood, poultry, and eggs are listed in the protein group without mention of pasture-raised, organic, or wild-caught vs. factory assembly-line cattle, veal, pork, poultry and eggs, even though the nutritional profile of the latter is far inferior. Even worse, commercially-raised cattle, pigs, poultry and farm-raised fish contain growth hormones, antibiotics and other drugs that humans should not ingest second-hand. And the often-times cruel-beyond-imagination and unsanitary conditions to which commercial livestock and farm-raised fish are subjected, should be reason enough to look for alternative protein sources, both animal and plant-based.

- Oils and fats quite often are all lumped together, usually as evil, "limit consumption"–type foods, neglecting the need for what is appropriately termed *"essential fats"*. The poorly understood (at the time) recommendation to switch to a low-fat diet was principally responsible for the exploding epidemic of obesity during the 80s. Another "F" grade for the government experts and all the food and diet industries that jumped on the bandwagon.

- Water and other liquids are usually missing entirely, and rarely is there a mention of such important health-related issues as breathing clean air, stress reduction, and physical activity.

- Also M.I.A.: herbs and spices. This, despite the universally recognized importance of including both in your diet for reasons ranging from better digestion to cancer-fighting properties, beneficial effects on many diseases, and powerful preventive health agents. Drug companies, however, have figured it out. They distill the most powerful compounds of natural herbs, plants, and even tree bark and then sell us the resulting pills or potions (less effective than the "real thing") at huge profit margins.

We can – and must – do better than that, and rather than burying vital-for-life foods and liquids in yet another burial chamber, I feel they are better off in a life-saving ark. My **"Food Ark"**™ has not been co-designed by powerful food lobbies nor does it cower to perceived "necessities" (aka protecting the established fast-food and food-processing industrial complex). Instead it only has one uncompromising goal: attaining and maintaining good health.

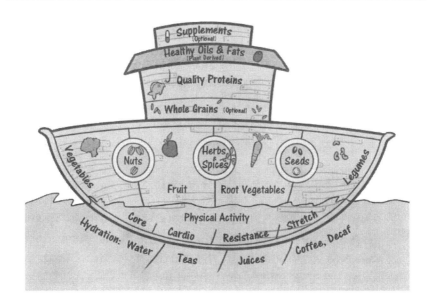

WHAT THEN ARE SAFE AND HEALTHY FOODS WITHIN THE VARIOUS FOOD GROUPS OF THE FOOD ARK™?

Proteins
- Wild caught fish (fresh preferred, but including frozen and canned); some "responsibly" farmed fish may be O.K. – check on a case-by-case basis
- Organic eggs from *pasture-raised* poultry (better than "cage-free" or "free-range" – these definitions have loopholes large enough for entire egg factories to slip through)
- Venison
- Buffalo
- Game
- *Organic, pasture-raised* poultry (again, better than cage-free or free-range)
- Organic, pasture-raised, 100% grass-fed lamb & beef
- Tofu & tempeh from non-GMO soy beans

Vegetables (organic and/or local-grown preferred)
- Green, leafy vegetables (spinach, collard-, mustard-, turnip greens, kale, some lettuces, etc.)
- Cruciferous vegetables (cabbages, broccoli, cauliflower, Brussels sprouts, etc.)
- Asparagus, bok choy, mushrooms, peppers**, avocados** and tomatoes**, eggplants, onions, garlic, cucumbers, green beans, squashes and zucchini, other local or ethnic vegetables.

(** technically fruit)

Fruit (organic and/or local-grown preferred)
- All berries, apples, oranges, bananas, papayas, mangos, plums, kiwi, pears, peaches, nectarines, apricots, melons, grapes, cherries, pomegranates, pineapple, persimmons, mangosteens, jack fruit, dragon fruit, passion fruit, and many other tropical fruit; dried fruit.

Root Vegetables (organic and/or local-grown preferred)
- Celery (the root, not the stalks), parsnip, carrot, sweet potato, yam, radishes (including daikons), rutabaga, turnip, beet, potato, burdock, taro, yucca, boniata, cassava, malanga, other ethnic varieties

Legumes* (organic and/or local-grown preferred)
- Beans, peas, peanuts, chickpeas, lentils

Nuts & Seeds* (organic preferred)
- Walnuts, almonds, pecans, cashew, Brazil, hazelnuts, pistachios, pine nuts
- Pumpkin seeds, sesame, sunflower, poppy, flax seeds (ground)

Essential Fatty Acids / Healthy Oils (organic preferred)
- Fish oil (naturally occurring in fish, or in pill form, or cod-liver oil; high in omega-3 fatty acids), flaxseed oil (highest in omega-3 f. a.) olive oil (highest in monounsaturated f.a.), macadamia nut oil (monounsaturated f.a.), walnut oil (high in omega-3 f.a.), avocado oil (high in monounsaturated f.a.), most other nut and seed oils, including, pumpkin, and tea seed oils. Use only moderate amounts of canola oil (monounsaturated & omega-3 f.a.; great for cooking), and peanut oil (monounsaturated f.a.; great for cooking). Also, small amounts of saturated fats are O.K., as they occur naturally in plant-based oils (including tropical oils), nuts, seeds, and in organic meats, eggs, etc. "Earth Balance"™ puts out a decent "butter-like" spread, but naturally occurring fats as listed above are preferable. Healthy, but "a little goes a long way": sesame oil (too high in omega-6). One more word about flaxseed oil: the "L & G" research now claims that it could be bad for us! Why, it may raise the level of anti-oxidants in our bodies! Come to think of it, so does exercise. My take on this: until more convincing arguments appear on the scene enjoy that source of omega-3 fatty acids, as always in moderation.

- The surprising news about animal fats: not all saturated fats are created equal … and there's more to the black-and-white "bad" LDL cholesterol vs. "good" HDL cholesterol theory. For one, increased intake of cholesterol-containing foods will not automatically raise blood cholesterol levels in most healthy people. Typically the body would respond by manufacturing less of its own cholesterol. Further complicating matters is new scientific evidence suggesting the existence of four different types of LDL cholesterol, and not all of them may be "bad" – but the smallest, densest forms of LDL ("very small LDL" and "small LDL" are the non-creative terms right now) seem to pose the biggest threat to one's health. How to avoid them? The science is still out, but as usual it's not as easy as "eat this / don't eat that", especially since testing for these sub-classes of LDL cholesterol is not widely available yet. One thing seems to be sure though: keeping one's weight in the "healthy" range is the best strategy to reduce <u>all</u> forms of LDL, so worry less about fats in general (read: *consume normal amounts*), keep the intake of <u>refined</u> carbohydrates low (zero would be just fine), and get or stay active. Sorry to say, all the new wisdoms we gain about cholesterol and fats still do not represent a carte blanche to consume excess amounts of fats – or carbs for that matter.
- <u>Oils to avoid:</u> cottonseed oil (the worst of the bunch), and most vegetable oils, like safflower, sunflower, corn, soy, generic "vegetable blends" (they are usually of lower quality, and disproportionably high in omega-6 f.a.), all margarines containing transfats, partially or fully hydrogenated fats, any type of "shortening". Think *"Inflammatory Foods"* and skip them, or keep consumption to a minimum.

Common Herbs (organic and/or local-grown preferred);
- Basil, thyme, marjoram, sage, dill, rosemary, laurel leaf, parsley, cilantro, coriander leaves, ginger, chili peppers, curry leaves, mint, bay leaves, oregano, chives, lemongrass, kaffir

leaves, pandan leaves (screw pine), tarragon, purslane, other ethnic herbs

Common Spices (organic preferred – or grow your own!)
- Turmeric, curry, paprika, pepper, chili powder, allspice, saffron, anise, cumin, caraway seeds, clove, cinnamon, nutmeg, cardamom, cayenne, mustard seed, celery seeds, ginger, garlic, fennel, file gumbo, horseradish, licorice, vanilla, other ethnic spices

---

Optional: Whole Grains (organic)
- Gluten-Free preferred: brown (unpolished) rice, millet, buckwheat, quinoa, teff, amaranth (not technically a grain), corn, sorghum; possibly oats (status disputed)
- Gluten-containing: wheat, rye, barley; possibly oats (status disputed)

---

* **NOTE:** the amino acids of **legumes & nuts** or **legumes & seeds** or **legumes & whole grains** complement each other to form complete (plant-based) proteins

---

What's conspicuously missing in the Food Ark™? *Inflammatory Foods* that the human species would be better off doing without – read on.

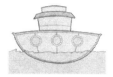

WHAT – NO DAIRY PRODUCTS?

That's right: **you don't <u>need</u> dairy products at all**, apart from mother's milk for infants. As a matter of fact humans were originally designed to become dairy-intolerant after being weaned from mother's milk in infancy. Only when this gene was switched off in Northern Europeans (giving them a much better chance of survival with the addition of a readily available source of protein) did milk and dairy products become part of the human diet. My suggestion: if you are at the verge of starving – like when an earthquake traps you in a supermarket dairy aisle - go ahead and drink up. Otherwise your body will be just fine without it – and chances are it will be a lot healthier in the process.

Don't take my word for it? Go ahead and eliminate dairy products from your diet for 2-3 weeks, and replace with enriched almond milk, rice milk, non-GMO soy milk, and/or coconut milk–based "yoghurt" (and keep up your variety of vegetables, fruit & healthy proteins). I bet you'll feel better – and you just improved the quality of your life and you may just stick with the healthier dairy-free lifestyle. Suffice it to say that our bodies – many of which are lactose-intolerant – are trying to tell us something. And the myth about strong bones and osteoporosis-fighting dairy products is just that – a myth, kept alive no doubt by "interested parties". Consider this: the countries with the highest consumption of dairy products (the U.S., Scandinavian countries) also have the highest rates of osteoporosis cases. You will be better off with a diet rich in green, leafy vegetables, legumes, tofu, and a fair amount of exposure to the sun (vitamin "D"). And if you feel you must supplement for optimum health, calcium supplements (with magnesium) and fortified almond or rice or soy milks will furnish calcium without the added "baggage" of saturated fats and too much animal protein, not to mention drug residues, antibiotics, growth hormones, etc.

<u>Best dairy product to avoid</u>: cheese. Not surprisingly it is also one of the most highly advertised foods, yet is thin on health benefits (there's better ways to get your calcium, and much better protein

sources too), and overloaded with saturated fats to the point that it nearly manages to make plain old cow's milk look healthy in comparison. Ponder this: have you ever seen any athletes claim that their performance was due to a generous intake of cheese?

<u>Best dairy product to give the benefit of the doubt:</u> whey protein isolates. Maybe a million athletes from bodybuilders to Olympians to endurance athletes **can** be wrong, but this type of protein is generally regarded as ideally suited for muscular performance and recovery, and has an enviable track record in that respect. With no, or minimal lactose, chances are most people can tolerate whey protein isolates, and may want to consider adding this to their diet, especially if protein intake from other sources is low. People with severe lactose intolerance issues or strict vegetarians ("vegans") would be well advised to check with their healthcare professional prior to including any new food, especially dairy-based.

GRAINS ANYONE?

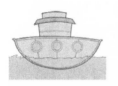 And why are grains given "optional" status in the "Food Ark™"? Because contrary to what we have been led to believe, **you don't need grains to lead a long and healthy, active life.** Heresy you say? Maybe so, and you won't hear this kind of advice from the US government or conventional wisdom nutrition experts. The cereal makers of the world, among others, will make sure of that. However some highly respected researchers have questioned the wisdom of mankind having adopted an agricultural lifestyle.

Mankind survived the toughest of circumstances for millions of years without cultivated grains. But, in the relatively short period since grain cultivation began (the past 10,000 years), we have been plagued by epidemics, food shortages, <u>new and/or more widespread diseases</u>, mass warfare, and the unhealthy accumulation of way too many people in confined spaces. (If you consider cities with populations of 15+ million success stories for mankind, you have probably never lived in one.) A good many of these civilization issues are the direct or indirect result of adopting grains as staples, partly due to their consumption, partly due to facilitating explosive population growth & straining the world's resources.

Still, I am not advocating eliminating all grains from your diet. A convincing argument can be made that after 10,000 or so years, mankind has adapted to the consumption of grains. People eating largely a grain-based diet have not become extinct (although they are burdened with many "civilization diseases"), and there are some nutritive qualities in **whole** grains that may go missing if people were to yank grains off the dinner plate <u>without making healthy adjustments</u>. There is also a very good possibility that by far the worst effects of grains in your diet are not so much the grains themselves but how we have leached most nutrients out of grains and processed what little remained to near-death. **We can, and should, however eliminate all processed white flour (and**

refined sugar) products. If nothing else, let's give **whole, gluten-free and non-genetically modified grains** the benefit of the doubt for the time being and let's assume that reasonable amounts (not 11 servings!) can contribute to a healthy diet.

Not convinced? Try the same approach to processed white flour products that you should take with dairy products. Exclude them, and all gluten-containing products, from your diet for 2-3 weeks and see how your body reacts. Chances are it will love it – and you'll reap the benefits! Feel worse after a few days? That could actually be a good sign of sugar withdrawal symptoms, and once you get beyond that, real improvements should be noticed. Are there any "good grains" that are worth keeping? Look no further than **brown (unpolished) rice, millet, buckwheat, quinoa, teff, amaranth** (not technically a grain), **corn, sorghum, and possibly oats** (gluten-free status disputed), all preferably **organic,** and all in **moderate quantities.** And since widely available whole grains combine with legumes to form a complete protein this is another good reason why it may not be desirable to eliminate whole grains altogether. Doing so could take us a step closer towards the dangerous **exclusionary diet.**

DRINK UP!

Don't forget the biggest part of your dietary intake: **water**, some of which is naturally contained in foods and some that needs to be consumed in the form of plain water, tea, coffee or juices. How much water (or liquid) is right for you? Forget about formulas thrown around like "Eight 8oz. cups of water a day" not including coffee. Those "one size fits all" rules are borderline worthless, except for the message that you should probably drink a lot. What's a lot for an 18-year old teenager cannot be the same as for a 50-something sedentary man, not taking into account the time of the year (temperature), diet, health status, weight, activity levels, and a long list of other factors. A rough rule of thumb would be to consume approx. 1 liter (approx. 34 ounces) of non-alcoholic beverages for every 1000 calories consumed <u>as a minimum,</u> resulting in approx. 2 liters for women and 2-1/2 liters for men. But you'll be better off forgetting about formulas and going with the more practical advice to drink throughout the day to the point where your urine is a pale yellow color (although vitamin supplements can darken that somewhat).

The good news? **Consuming a lot of liquids will flush out waste products in your body and help you lose weight!** Which liquids are best? In order of relative 'healthfulness', they are:

- Clean, filtered water is the gold standard. This should be your first "go-to" beverage in the morning to "wake up" your digestive system and to re-hydrate. As mentioned earlier, you may want to install a reverse-osmosis water filtration system at home. Compared to buying bottled water this will result in **big** <u>long-term $ savings</u>, not to mention that it is environmentally friendlier than clogging up our landfills with one-way plastic bottles. Any impurities that can be found in some municipal water will be filtered out by a 5-stage R.O. system; you'll never miss the smell of chlorine, trust me. Store filtered water in a glass container vs. anything 'plastic', to avoid possible contamination with ingredients that can leach from the plastic material.

- **Teas**, including **green tea** and **white tea** (decaf preferred) add a healthy variety to your liquid intake. The positive health effect of **tea**, especially **green tea,** has been researched extensively with impressive results. Traditionally used in China for centuries, green tea may play a role in weight loss, reducing heart disease risks, lowering cholesterol, increasing fat oxidation, lowering your chances to get certain cancers, and may even reduce your chances of contracting Alzheimer's disease, to mention just a few of its many purported benefits. You have nothing to lose by adding it to your life. Even though green tea has less caffeine that is also absorbed at a slower rate, I would still suggest using more naturally decaffeinated varieties, especially later in the day. **Black tea** too has beneficial properties (caffeine-free is better), but it can also interfere with the absorption of certain key minerals, like iron, so overall tea consumption should be heavily tilted towards (naturally decaffeinated) **green** or **white teas**. And you may want to re-think that traditional iced tea with your meal.

  And don't overlook **fruit teas, herb teas,** or **"dessert" teas**: they add variety to your liquid intake and are generally safe to consume in large quantities (except maybe "dieters tea" or other strong teas with reputed medicinal qualities). A properly prepared "dessert tea" (Vanilla Chai anyone, or Chocolate-Hazelnut?) with a dash of rice or almond milk may make you wonder why you ever spent upwards of $6.00 at your local "Mega-Bucks" for a less healthy coffee or tea concoction loaded with empty calories. You should be safe using tea brands like Bigelow, Stash, or Celestial Seasonings.

- **Juices** can be a healthy way to meet your daily liquid "quota", but excessive consumption can be problematic. Their biggest drawback is the **amount and type** of calories:

lots of them, and mostly simple carbs in the form of sugars. Drinking them just for thirst will overload your system on both accounts. However, <u>adding</u> a little bit to your diet can be a good thing – if 1<u>00% whole, unfiltered juices</u> are used ('just say no' to see-through clear juices) that are <u>mixed with water</u>. Try for a 50-50 ratio. Not enough taste left or not sweet enough? Cheat! Add a few drops of stevia, a packet of Truvia™, some xylitol, or a packet of 'yellow' or 'pink' if you must, and taste the difference. Tropicana™ does exactly the same thing: their "Trop 50" O.J. is mixed with water and a little bit of sucralose and voilà – it sells for the same price as 100% O.J. You can do better – at half the cost – at home. And ignore anything that says "juice drink" on the label – it's thinly veiled sugar water, no matter how many vitamins they add.

- What about **coffee**? A cup early in the day will probably not wreck your health, and coffee does have some beneficial effects. After that (one) cup it's probably best to stop, or at the very least switch to the naturally decaffeinated variety. But unless you have a strong addiction to coffee (it happens – a lot, so stick with decaf after your morning jolt), there is also no good reason to have it be a part of your fluid intake. "Coffee Deficiency Syndrome" was not a recognized medical condition last time I checked.

- **Sodas** do way more damage than good and shouldn't use up space in your refrigerator – or your body. Can't live without them? Sure you can, if your goal is a healthy, new "you". But as an interim 'crutch', at least make sure they don't contain any (empty) sugar calories (you want to lose weight and keep your teeth, don't you?), phosphoric acid (which attacks tooth enamel, as does citric acid to a lesser extent), sodium (which can kill when consumed in excess), or caffeine (face it - it's a drug, and the sooner you kick the habit the better. Your quality of sleep will improve too). Oh, and carbonated beverages will make the body retain fluids, never a good thing.

- Just when you thought we hit rock-bottom as far as unhealthy beverages are concerned, there is even worse out there: **energy drinks** - loaded with empty sugar calories, PLUS enough caffeine to wake the comatose, not to mention other ingredients of undetermined health properties. They are especially worrisome for teenagers or young adults, which sadly is one of the key demographic groups these drinks target. I used to consume my fair share of the sugar-free versions, and when I kicked the habit my quality of life (and sleep!) took a quantum leap for the better. There is ONE application where these "monster" drinks are actually good for you: when you have to drive beyond your bedtime – being a live "wired" person beats being a dead, previously-healthy person anytime. Of course not getting or staying behind the wheel when you get tired would be hugely better yet. O.K., there may be a second benefit to energy drinks, when used occasionally for competitive performance improvements. Keep in mind that the "kick-start" abilities of caffeine wear off with heavy use, so if you need that jolt of coffee first thing in the morning <u>every morning</u>, chances are it won't do much for you. <u>Not</u> drinking it will most likely result in withdrawal symptoms, which should be a wake-up call that you are addicted and that you should consider kicking the caffeine habit. Once you are over the withdrawal symptoms (less than a week) you'll feel better than ever.

So there you have it, the liquids of choice for your body, from best to worst. And since (healthy) <u>hydration</u> is the subject of this discourse I see no reason to include alcohol.

Footnote: <u>timing</u> is everything, and that holds true for fluid intake also. Sure, just consuming the right <u>amount</u> of liquids is the most critical consideration, but the issue of timing should not be overlooked. Your body usually is the most dehydrated first thing in the morning; hence we like to start our day with juice, or tea or coffee. This would be a good time to <u>re-hydrate, with water</u>

first (hopefully plain, filtered water), then juice (diluted with water), or tea, or coffee.

There are different schools of thought out there as far as drinking with meals is concerned. I side with the theory that drinking a lot of beverages (of any kind) with meals is generally not a good idea. Sure, a small amount of liquid (1 cup maybe) can be a good thing, but drinking lots of iced tea (free re-fills of that 24oz cup?) or other beverages with your meal will have your meal float in a stomach with diluted digestive acid way longer than it should. And you might feel uncomfortably full, with food and liquid sloshing around. Not drinking 30-60 minutes prior to a meal, and not again for 1-2 hours after a normal-sized meal works best for me, but you may want to experiment with the timing that feels just right for you.

WHAT ABOUT SUPPLEMENTS?

Now THERE is a topic that generates a lot of heated arguments. Many books have been written on this subject, and I do not intend to add to that list – or discuss the pros and cons of taking supplements at great lengths. But I think supplements can be included as part of a healthy diet & lifestyle for several reasons.

First off they are called "supplements" for a reason. They are not "replacements" for skipped vegetables or fruits or quality proteins or fats, or an otherwise deficient diet. Stop for a moment and let this sink in.

One good reason to consider supplementing even a healthy diet is the fact, that while the human body's requirements for nutrients such as vitamins & minerals probably has not changed over the eons, increased stress and pollution alone may require **higher** intakes. Plus, it is a sad fact that cultivating ever decreasing varieties of fewer vegetables and fruits in depleted, exhausted soils has resulted in <u>measurably lower vitamin & mineral contents.</u> If you were to look at, say, a conventionally grown apple of today and compare it to an apple grown 50 or more years ago, chances are you may only be getting 80 or 70 percent of the apple's nutrients of yesteryear. So you are getting a bigger serving of 'empty' calories and less nutritional value.

Also, it has been suggested that the saying "you are what you eat" should be amended to sound more like "you are what you <u>absorb</u> from what you eat". It is generally accepted that absorption of nutrients decreases with age, although a good part of that is more a matter of decreasing activity than increasing age. Still, in general, we absorb less vital nutrients from food as we age. This probably happens after humans reach their physical peak in the mid-twenties, and continues well into old age. At age 40, when the realization starts to sink in that we may not, after all, be immortal, it might be a good idea to try to do something about this reduced absorption of nutrients from food. Starting earlier than that will probably do no harm, and of course it's never too late to start, but somewhere in that general age category it might be a good idea to try to make sure we get all the bang for our buck from the food we eat. Therefore some **digestive enzymes** as simple as papaya extract, or more potent natural digestive aids should be the first "supplement" to be considered. (And no, antacids do not qualify. See your doctor if you are unsure if and how to get started.) Usually taken with meals, you may want to start by adding quality enzymes to dinners, when digestion is slower and less efficient than earlier during the day. "More" is usually not "better", so it would be prudent never to exceed manufacturers' recommendations. Bonus: some enzymes may reduce muscle inflammation after intense exercise.

Also, it is generally accepted that a daily **multi-vitamin/mineral supplement** is a healthy addition to the adult diet and at the very least won't do any harm. There is considerably less agreement as to what types or brands of supplements are best, with some advocating that all supplements are pretty much the same and strictly buying by price is O.K., while others insist that only the way to go is with top-tier (expensive) brands. Since I don't believe in the "lowest-bidder-is-best" theory in anything in life, sticking with established, reputable companies is probably the smart thing to do and then let price influence your final decision. And since the recommended dosage for calcium would result in horse pill–sized tablet or capsule, a separate **calcium supplement** is usually recommended also.

And one thing leads to another … so if you take additional calcium supplements make sure you also get adequate amounts of **magnesium**, without which calcium absorption is poor at best, and can result in a dangerous mineral imbalance. Ditto for **vitamin "D"**, the "sunshine vitamin" – without adequate amounts of it, your body's absorption of calcium is poor (this may partly explain the paradox of high calcium intake in this country, and sky-high numbers of osteoporosis cases). Luckily many calcium supplements are available these days with magnesium and vitamin "D" added. And all these fat-soluble vitamins need – you guessed it – fat in the diet to be properly absorbed, another stake through the low-fat / no-fat diet craze. Another good reason to add a daily multi to your diet is vitamin B12. Vegetarians especially may often have low intake and absorption rates, and this vitamin is also crucial for older people suffering from gastritis and to ward off pernicious anemia.

How about **vitamin "C"** supplements – should you take them? There too, qualified scientists have been tossing arguments (and mud) around for a long time, with some saying it will prevent (or cure) the common cold, while others say it will only result in expensive urine. To the best of my knowledge though, consuming "normal" quantities of vitamin "C" has never been linked with any health concerns. It is considered a rather benign substance (again, when not taken in huge excess quantities), **and** this water-soluble vitamin is excreted readily from your body. Therefore, I don't see much harm in making sure you get enough vitamin "C" in supplement form **above and beyond** (not "instead" of) your dietary intake. Check your multi vitamin/mineral supplement, and add vitamin "C" if deemed necessary. I have taken rather large doses of vitamin "C" (among other supplements) and some-times go years without catching a cold. Other factors are most likely at play also, but I consider additional "C" intake a cheap insurance policy to avoid most colds and maybe some other infec-tious diseases.

Adding individual vitamin and/or mineral supplements to your diet is treacherous territory, and you are well advised to check with your health care professional before "self-prescribing" such supplements. Iron supplementation would be a prime example of the "don't try this at home without medical advice" category. There are however some supplements that have received a lot of attention lately, usually for good reasons, so I feel I should men-tion them.

- **Vitamin "D":** the stealth vitamin no longer. More and more nutrition experts have cautiously agreed there seems to be a vitamin "D" deficiency among most Americans. Made by the human body when skin is exposed to sunlight (and contained in some foods) most people don't get enough of this "sunshine vitamin" (which is actually a hormone). Vitamin "D" is crucial for proper calcium absorption and mineral balance in the human body, among other things. Sedentary and/or indoor lifestyles and skin-cancer scares having everybody applying layers of sun-block creams will do that to you. (And speaking of sedentary: excess body fat reduces blood levels of vitamin D). Nobody seems to agree what "safe" levels of supplementation are (when justified), but the dosages seem to go up with every scientific study. Stay up-to-date on the latest, always-changing recommendations and don't exceed manufacturers' recommended dosages.

Actually, the evolving story of vitamin "D" requirements is a good example of just how much confusion is "out there" – in the scientific community and the general public. Since "D" is a fat-soluble vitamin it is considered to have the potential of causing toxicity in large doses (this holds true for all fat-soluble vitamins – A,D,E,K), and the low recommended daily value is 200 I.U. (International Units). More and more research points to much higher levels being necessary for good health, with some credible sources now suggesting 1000-2000 Int. Units – a tenfold increase! Yet there are many reputable manufacturers that sell vitamin "D" supplements in local grocery & drug stores in 5000 I.U. strengths! Who are we supposed to believe? I have no intention of wading into this controversy; what works for me is not necessarily good for anybody else. All I can recommend is, do your research, consult with your doctor, and then make your decisions. The best way to obtain enough vitamin "D": moderate exposure to sunlight (10-15 minutes a day, 2-3 times per week; most healthy people can handle that much exposure without sunscreen). Can't beat Mother Nature, but avoid too much sun exposure for the well-known skin cancer link. One thing everybody seems to agree on: <u>we need more vitamin "D" as we get older.</u> And as usual – more is not better, as over-supplementation carries health risks. (Consider this: Mega-doses of vitamin "D" are used in some rat poisons.) The good news: excessive exposure to sunshine does not lead to vitamin "D" toxicity.

- **Glucosamine-Chondroitin-MSM**: are they the miracle cure for achy, aging joints – or so much snake oil? Who knows, but the consensus seems to be that they don't do any harm if taken as recommended by the manufacturers. Many people swear by them, so if you experience pain in your joints you may want to experiment with them and see if they do the trick for you.

- **Fish Oil / Omega-3 / flaxseed oil supplements**: the typical Western Diet is top-heavy with omega-6, at the expense of omega-3 fatty acids. These higher levels of omega-6 fatty acids may be linked to cardiovascular diseases, diabetes, hypertension, obesity, inflammatory diseases (such as rheumatoid arthritis) and some types of cancers. One way to reverse that unhealthy trend is to supplement with these nutrients. A better way would be to reduce the intake of omega-6 fatty acids, and include several servings of fatty fish (salmon, sardines, herring, mackerel, tuna, swordfish, haddock, halibut, etc.) in your diet (2-3 per week as a bare minimum), and add (ground) **flax seeds** (keep frozen) and/or **flaxseed oil** (keep refrigerated) to your diet. And you would do well to replace c.c. eggs (4:19 ratio of omega-3 vs. omega-6!) with pasture-raised eggs (3:1 ratio of omega-3 vs. omega-6!), and farm-raised fish (2:1 "3" vs. "6") with wild-caught fish (7:1 "3" vs. "6"), although exact ratios may vary depending on species and other factors. Again, these supplements are generally considered safe, so you may want to add them to your diet in the recommended dosages, although natural sources should be your first line of defense. **Oils to avoid** (or greatly limit consumption), mainly due to their high omega-6 content: animal fats, red meat, dairy products, and oils from soybeans, corn, sesame seeds, wheat germ, safflowers, and the worst offender of all "vegetable oils" – cottonseed oil.

- **Active cultures**: found in fermented foods, with yoghurt (milk or soy or coconut – based) being the most visible / advertised option. The health benefits derived from "friendly intestinal bacteria" are pretty much universally embraced, so taking supplements can be an acceptable means to get all the live cultures necessary for good health. And supplementing with active cultures is generally <u>recommended</u> when taking antibiotics. As usual, getting these beneficial active cultures is best achieved by eating the foods that contain them, which also include kimchi, sauerkraut, miso, and tempeh.

- **Protein supplements / Amino Acids**: <u>they are not just for body builders anymore!</u> In light of the fact that protein absorption rates decline with age, coupled with natural loss of muscle mass (age-related, but even more due to diminished activity levels), older adults especially should avail themselves of this muscle "keeper". As should anybody embarking on a serious exercise program, when immediate post-workout consumption of quality protein calories, in conjunction with carbohydrates, is <u>crucial</u>. No need to "get ripped" with 300-calorie per serving hardcore weight-lifters' supplements, on top of your usual foods. A 100-200 calorie per serving high-protein supplement (usually containing whey) such as EAS Myoplex™ or Muscle Milk™ or one of several of the AMP product line from GNC immediately after intense or long exercise will jump-start the recovery process and result in performance gains, rather than chronic fatigue. Casein proteins too will aid in the recovery process (especially when taken in the evening). These dairy-based supplements should be regarded as an imperfect compromise, but have the advantage of being widely available. Animal-free protein formulas (rice, pea, mixed vegetable, and non-GMO soy protein isolates) or those made from organic eggs would be better choices, so shop around to find the supplemental protein source of your choice, and "mix-and-match" for best results.

Not working out, but still want to increase your protein intake without adding too many calories, such as people on a calorie-restricted diet? Include the occasional protein shake in your diet (as a *supplement*, or a rare meal replacement, not in addition to all other foods you consume in a day). Another easy way to up your protein intake (and eliminate a highly unhealthy food-type substance at the same time) would be to add protein supplements in powder form (or ready-to-drink shakes) instead of non-dairy creamer to your decaf coffee or tea. This will safely raise your intake of easily absorbed quality protein.

Another way to add quality amino acids (the building blocks of protein) is in pill form. There are hundreds of products out there, and sifting through them can be daunting. I have had good success with Twin Lab Amino Fuel 1000 ("Mega Mass"). Don't be scared off by the words "bodybuilding amino acids" on the label. I have been taking them for a long time and kept my runner's physique - nobody has mistaken me for Arnie yet. "GNC Amino Burst 3000" is another good option. I suspect that protein supplementation for the aging population is one of the best health-improving steps they can take, and will go "mainstream" in the coming years. As always, check with your doctor first before embarking on any supplementation program. Also, in the case of protein shakes, the recommended dosages are usually targeted to hardcore users in their prime (plus, the manufacturers have a financial interest in selling you a lot of it), so they need to be scaled back considerably for most everybody else.

- **Resveratrol:** It is the "Wonder Drug of the Century" (!) … "promotes longer and healthier life" … "has powerful anti-aging and cancer-fighting properties" … "can improve athletic performance by 100%" ... "is a strong anti-oxidant" ... "has antiviral and anti-inflammatory benefits" - the list of wild health benefits goes on and on.

So maybe this really is the mythical "fountain-of-youth-in-a-pill" ... but you may want to google "resveratrol side effects" first before you order a case of the stuff. For one, the "proven" longer life spans only seem to apply to fruit flies, worms and yeast, and doubling of athletic performance gives bragging rights to mice on their tiny treadmills only. And it seems like the (100 %!) endurance gains obtained with lab animals for example can come with a price of athletic injuries in non-rodents such as humans. Anecdotal evidence is mounting that athletes using resveratrol in supplement form come down with mysterious Achilles tendonitis, plantar fasciitis, calf muscle and possibly other injuries that make any claimed "athletic performance improvements" a moot point. Now we all know that "anecdotal evidence" ranks just a tad higher in scientific credibility than reading tea leaves ... but when "somebody" incurs 3 calf muscle injuries in the span of nine weeks after not having had any "issues" in that area during the previous 20-plus years of running (and no more since discontinuing taking said supplement), then maybe there's something to this particular "anecdotal evidence".

Bottom Line: eat all the grapes you want (which are high in resveratrol) but if your goal is improved athletic performance keep in mind that you are not a little mousy in a lab. As for all the other healths claims "out there" – for resveratrol <u>and all other new miracle supplements</u> - google for side effects and <u>see your doctor first</u>, then decide for yourself.

THE PLAN

Remember those old-timer immigrant stories, or movie scripts, about the new-to-town stranger, usually young and naïve, stepping off the train (or plane, or ship) from a different city (or country)? He or she arrives, walks around, suitcase in hand, curiously tries to get oriented in the new environment, wondering what this 'new world' will hold for him or her. Fast-forward 24 hours and the suitcase and all the money are gone with the nice-seeming 'friend' who offered to help the new arrivée get settled in but, instead, left the naïve newcomer with a painful lesson and not much else. (BTW, this sort of thing still happens in other parts of the world today.)

Does that sound like YOU?

"No way", you say. *"How naïve do you think I am?* **"Laughable".**

As much as I hate to disillusion you, if you are overweight or obese, chances are very good that **this is <u>you</u> 100%. Every day of your life.** No, not stepping off a train, wide-eyed - but starting every new day without a plan as to *what* foods you will eat, *how much* you will eat, *when* you will eat them, and what – if any - physical activity you will participate in. And without a firm plan that puts determination and confidence into your step, and a healthy structure into your life, you fall prey to nice "friends" – fast food outlets, restaurants, office snacks, soda machines, birthday cakes at the office, candy bar machines, and – eventually – the recliner at home. Your decisions are guided by the worst advisors you can think of – an empty stomach and "first-available" choices. Don't believe it – try walking into a bakery or deli with an empty stomach. **You are doomed to fail** – and repeat the same mistake over and over again. You know there has to be a better way – **but you have to plan for it.**

Instead of the above scenario, imagine that new arrivista having planned his trip, stepping into the new city with a trusted contact to meet, knowing how to get there, and knowing what to do upon getting there. There is focus, determination, and purpose emanating from that person and any scamster who approaches is confidently ignored. They don't have a chance.

That is the person you want to be.

So how do you get there?

You wouldn't go into a business meeting without a plan, based on the "homework" you did. You wouldn't just jump in the car to go to a party without a map and/or knowing how to get there. You wouldn't leave the house without having planned what to wear, according to the weather and the purpose of your trip. **And you shouldn't wake up in the morning without a plan for 3 square meals, 2 snacks, good beverage options, and a plan for some physical activity.**

If you don't want to fall prey to tempting "first-available" calories you have to plan every single meal. "And who has time for that?" you say? Not an acceptable excuse in the land where adults find time to spend 3-5 hours on average a day sitting in front of the TV and 18 hours a week online! Especially since a lot of that planning doesn't take any time at all – you can plan your meals and workouts for the next day while commuting, during exercise, during your lunch – maybe even during that boring business meeting. There you go – you can formulate a plan without spending any "real" time on it. Yes, you do have to follow through with your plan, and that will take a <u>little</u> more time than living life "happy-go-lucky" – which has gotten you into all this trouble in the first place. Can you "sacrifice" a half hour or so from your busy TV (or Facebook schedule) in return for a healthier you? For feeling great all day long, day in – day out? I bet you can.

Here is what a typical day in the typical "average" person looks like (remember – being overweight is "average" these days).

- **"Average Joe"** had a long day in the office, and is on his way home. He is not hungry since he had a huge lunch with his buddies at the local "Cheap-Calories-Are-Us" restaurant. So he checks the mail, fires up the computer, or plays with the kids, or runs some errands, and eventually plops himself in front of the TV – or the computer.

- Dinner is pushed out to 8:00PM or later – and by then Joe is hungry again. So hungry as a matter of fact that he overeats at the worst time of the day, when his metabolism has started to retire for the day. Having that big steak probably wasn't a good idea this late in the day. Feeling way too full to go to bed anytime soon, Joe does his share to raise the national average of TV-watching time to 3-5 hours a day, although he snoozes through most of the last show. The thought of getting up early the next day to exercise – or plan and fix meals and snacks for the next day is D.O.A.

- The next morning it's time for breakfast – except Joe's dinner has not made a lot of progress since last night. A quick cup of coffee will do just fine – and it will help him "get started".

- It's mid-morning in the office and dinner did finally digest. With his metabolism at its peak, Joe's stomach starts to growl. No way will he make it until lunch hour. Not having brought any snacks he becomes a victim, ahem, "customer" of the office snack-vending machine or finds the donuts left over from the sales meeting. Joe digs in.

- Finally it's lunch time. Not liking to "brown-bag" it, Joe goes out with his pals again. The food smells good, and why should he waste those French fries that he paid for? Now he feels good again – until that mid-afternoon freight train laden with all those processed grease calories hits him square on. Eventually he rights himself and makes it through the rest of the day. Thank goodness there wasn't an afternoon meeting scheduled.

- Joe heads home again, not the least bit hungry …… and the same story repeats itself, again, and again.

Here is what a day in the life of **"Smarter-Than-Average-Jane"** looks like:

- Before dinner Jane takes a brisk 30-minute walk in her neighborhood. Her day in the office was a pressure-cooker, again, so this walk is a great stress reliever. Re-energized she has a small, early dinner, and then gets ready for the next day:
- Clothes, and a small snack ready for a short pre-breakfast cardio session: check
- Breakfast all planned: check
- 2 small snacks and a lunch packed: check
- Workout clothes and spare snacks packed for post-work weight-room session packed: check
- Jane skips TV and gets an early night in – she knows from experience that getting out of bed early for that pre-breakfast workout is a lot harder if she doesn't get enough sleep
- When the alarm goes off Jane is ready. Mind you, not like she'd want to uproot trees, but good enough to get out of bed and get going. Powered by a couple of slices of organic sweet potato topped with walnuts, natural peanut butter and a date she feels a whole lot better after her cardio session: 30 minutes of spinning, some of it at a high intensity, sipping water. (**Now** she is ready for those trees!)
- Breakfast tastes good (a cup of blueberry green tea, a hard-boiled egg, a slice of brown rice bread, natural peanut butter, and a whole orange), but Jane resists the temptation for second servings. For one, there are none – she only prepared a reasonably-sized meal, and for another, she knows that a small snack is waiting for her, mid-morning. Bonus: that box of donuts in the office doesn't look nearly as good as her snack (fresh strawberries and a small bag of mixed nuts, raisins and peanuts), so she is not even tempted. She also sips water throughout the day, or has an occasional cup of decaf green tea.
- For lunch Jane has her reasonably portioned home-made meal in the office lunch room (stir-fried veggies with curry

tofu). She knows better than eating too much and then fighting to stay awake (forget about being productive) by mid-afternoon. Since she doesn't spend half of her lunch time fighting traffic, finding a parking space, and waiting for her (inferior) lunch to arrive, Jane even has time to take a walk outside, and stocks up on her sunshine vitamin ("D").

- Sure enough, she avoids the blood-sugar roller coaster and even needs that mid-afternoon snack (veggie chips and a little hummus-flaxseed-sage dip) to power her through the post-work weight-room workout, sipping water throughout. A small, high-protein snack (EAS AdvantEDGE Carb Control™ shake: 110 cal. / 17g protein / 3 g fat) right after her workout starts the muscle repair job immediately, and will leave her less ravenous for dinner (a small piece of wild-caught soy-glazed salmon with rosemary wild rice, and steamed asparagus). This is just as well, because Jane steps on the scale every morning, first thing, and she 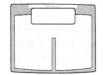 doesn't like 'omg surprises'. And waking up hungry for that first snack, or breakfast, is a great way to start the day.

- Time to get ready for the next day ..... a 30-minutes-or-so small investment in feeling great all day, day after day.

Guess who feels better all day, has more energy, fewer guilt trips, and overall better quality (and eventually *quantity*) of life? Jane is in control of her life and well-being, while Joe feels sluggish, has health readings of a man 20 years older than his birth certificate says, and is an easy target for fast-food advertising and empty calorie snacking. And chances are he'll meet a friendly heart surgeon soon.

So how do you get closer to resembling "Healthy Jane", rather than "Heart-Attack-Waiting-To-Happen-Joe"?

STEP 1: you have to make the mental "SWITCH" to commit to healthy, minimally processed "real" foods

Many processed foods have the 3 built-in, cheap "addictors": sugar, sodium, fat. These food-like substances have been "engineered" with great effort to get you addicted to them! That means your body craves more of these inferior "food" calories than it needs, something that is much less likely to happen with the "real", minimally processed food the human body has thrived on for millions of years. Worse yet, these "empty calories" don't fool the body, which still demands full servings of all the vital-for-life (and healthy) ingredients, so it asks for this nutrient-deficit to be erased. If we oblige and feed it low concentrations of quality ingredients surrounded by cheap and calorie-rich, but nutrient-poor 'packaging' (flavor enhancers) that may not signal the brain to stop the feeding frenzy – and the result isn't pretty. Let me illustrate this critical point by comparing fresh, organic apples to apple pie.

APPLE (approx. the same weight as apple pie) vs. APPLE PIE (1 slice)

	APPLE	APPLE PIE (1 slice)
Calories:	<100	410
Cholesterol:	0	150
Total Fat:	0.3g	16g
Vitamin C:	7.8mg	0
Sodium:	1mg	482mg
Fiber:	1.05g	0.6g

Still surprised why a plain apple scores a '96' on the food ratings chart and apple pie rates a '2'?

I don't want to be the grinch that stole your apple pie (there is a time and a place for apple pie, occasionally), but if you repeat this dietary intake pattern across the board (highly processed vs. unprocessed, whole) you can see how your meals will fall far short of nourishing your body. Hence the saying that is so typical of most Americans – "overfed and undernourished".

The first thing that may enter your mind when considering embarking on a major lifestyle change like that will be "but, but ... I can't possibly live without [.....]" – insert your favorite processed food(s). So *the first reaction is to think of nothing else but that food* (or type of foods), *to the point of obsession* about that great tragic loss in your life. Come on now – it's just a donut! Or fettuccini Alfredo! Or a burger! You have just set yourself up for failure, and the constant thinking about that – and other – "forbidden fruit" will sabotage any realistic chance of making a long-lasting change. <u>Instead, think exclusively of all the healthy foods you will have more of</u>, since you eliminated this – and other – unhealthy foods. Think crisp apples, roasted nuts, sweet potatoes, ripe tomatoes, rich avocados, wild-caught salmon, crunchy-fresh cucumber salad, real eggs, and so on. Stay in that "window" (or – better yet - don't think about food at all!), and close down the other "window" that has all the empty-calorie foods in it. Think about what you GAIN, not about what you LOSE.

<u>Don't become (or remain) a victim of the fast-food / industrial food complex (again!).</u> They have made cheap food-like items addictive in nature, and cast a wide net with availability of their "wares" all around you, 24/7. They softened up your resistance, weak as it may have been to start with, by targeted, deadly-effective advertising. They took away your natural ability to recognize what kinds of foods your body really needs, how much to have, and your capacity to say "when" you have had enough. **You should be angry**, for they have disassociated you from a healthy relationship with healthy foods and are a major reason for the obesity epidemic in this country, which we so successfully export around the world. It is time to declare your independence again – **you are not going to take it anymore. Start your own diet revolution now!**

(How guilty is the fast-food / processed food industrial complex? Let's just say that they saw fit to "influence" our upstanding lawmakers to pass the "Cheeseburger Bill", shielding them from lawsuits from obese individuals. Are we hitting a raw nerve there?)

<u>Don't become a casualty</u> – like so many deer.

"Let's go down to that corn feeder", says "Deer 1" to "Deer 2". "I don't know about that", says"Deer-2". "It seems too easy, and we never used to eat corn. It tastes great, but I always feel sluggish afterwards. And it gives me gas." "Deer-1" will have none of that. "I am going down there – I can taste that sweet corn already! See you later, worry-wart." Except," Deer-1" was never heard of again. Yup, it was opening day of deer hunting season.

No, they don't fatten you up with junk food and shoot you, but the final outcome is the same for humans. You fall for the "easy" calories, and premature death from preventable diseases is an all-but-certain outcome. You don't realize it, but **you are committing suicide with a knife and fork** (or a spoon, or chop sticks). Worse yet, unlike the hapless deer, you'll be picked clean first by ever-mounting health-care bills, money spent on ineffective miracle diets, and probably fall prey to other health-promising scams.

Still not convinced you can live without "that" food? Try this trick: surely you can live without it for, say a day or two, or 1-2 weeks – hopefully longer. Something curious will happen: the longer you make do without that unhealthy food item, the fewer cravings you will have for it – and you might just feel better too. **We develop the most addictive cravings for foods that we have often** and the addiction feeds on itself in a vicious circle. Once you break that cycle for a sufficiently long time the craving diminishes. I'll admit to some pretty unhealthy dietary habits in my past, until I was lucky to be introduced to the 'World's Best Dental Technician' (O.K., my subjective judgment). She convinced me that maybe living without caramel corn (and other sugary snacks) would be a sacrifice I could live with in return for not losing my teeth in the next few years. Yup, she scared me into becoming a healthier person. Eventually (much later) I did 'reward' myself at one time with some caramel corn again, and guess what: I had so looked forward to that small indulgence, yet ended up thoroughly disappointed. I had a "what was <u>that</u> all about" experience. It tasted good, but was totally unexciting. I never did finish that bag. Same with cheese, most meats, croissants, white pasta, pastries, chocolate, all sugars and sugar-loaded "treats", and a long list of other 'must-have' foods – once you eliminate all the inferior-quality calories, the cravings for them eventually disappear. And you'll discover that whole, minimally processed foods taste so much better! And if you feel like having that *occasional* treat – well, life isn't a "zero-tolerance" world. Don't deny yourself occasional tastes of new foods (especially when traveling abroad) or familiar treats (childhood favorites when visiting home). As long as the impact on overall calories consumed is largely negligible you're O.K.

STEP 2: you have to have all the healthy "real" foods available in your house if you want to embark on a healthy lifestyle

Let's go shopping. Following the guidelines for what foods you should eat (see "The Basics" chapter) you have to grocery-shop with a purpose, undistracted by special offers, appetizing-looking choices that are poor in nutritional value, and with a healthy disdain for reading lengthy ingredient lists indicative of how much processing has gone into that food. It has been said that your best supermarket strategy is to shop the "perimeters" only, and avoid the center aisles altogether. Good advice – as long as you know when and where to make exceptions. Trust me, if the majority of shoppers followed that old wisdom a lot of processed (spelled p r o f i t a b l e) foods would relocate next to vegetables and the fish counter. Oh, and just because meats are usually sold on the perimeter of the supermarkets doesn't mean that all's fair and good there – far from it. And of course some healthy, wholesome foods do reside in the aisles – 100% juices (use in moderation), dried fruit, natural peanut butter (among lots of not-so-healthy processed varieties), nuts, healthy oils, spices & dried herbs, canned beans (go for 'low sodium' varieties), etc.

So yes, compile that old-fashioned grocery list, then march into battle with a plan, and don't deviate from it. A better strategy than the old shop-the-perimeters system: if it has an ingredient list and is highly advertised, avoid it – or study it very carefully and eliminate highly processed "foods" with lengthy ingredient lists. You can live without that pint of umlaut ice cream. Or those whole-some-*looking* crackers (first ingredient: unbleached white flour …). Or that cereal with health claims jumping off the package (and tons of white sugar in the small print). Or that incredibly delicious-smelling rotisserie c.c. chicken (over 50% of supermarket chicken has salmonella or other bacteria). Or those empty-calorie soft drinks.

Your best defense against all those temptations is not buying anything that is unhealthy, over-processed, or otherwise not known for possessing any benefits for human health. Just purchase "approved" foods (see "The Basics" chapter) that you will need to prepare the meals for the next day (or more) and skip the "discretionary calories". Chances are you have plenty of those at home, and you may want to give serious thought to disposing of them to make room for your new choices. I abhor waste, yet you may be better off without some manufactured items masquerading as food in your home. You have to decide what is best for your health and your conscience and make those decisions. One way or another, sooner or later, most, if not all poor food choices should have cleared out of your life, and you will only have good choices available in your home. Sure, you can let that pint of premium umlaut ice-cream die of freezer burn, but chances are you might hear it calling you at midnight sooner or later, jeopardizing your dedication. So, eliminate all the questionable calories that have accumulated in your fridge, freezer, and pantry, and start with a clean slate. (I suggest that you minimize waste by donating non-perishable foods to organizations that assist the less fortunate – most of whom will be better off with less-than-perfect calories than no calories at all.)

Another advantage to having a well-stocked pantry and refrigerator at home: you are more likely to just walk past that tempting display of pastries or other less-than-wholesome foods in super-markets, convenience stores, bakeries, etc., <u>knowing that you have much better-for-you (and better tasting) food waiting for you at home.</u>

STEP 3: you have to know when to say "when" – and put down that fork

Easy for me to say, adhering to an exercise schedule that many professional athletes don't follow (who said baseball players?). Wrong: after every endurance competition my weight creeps up – until I make that mental "switch" and get back on track to lose those extra 5 lbs. or more, before the 5 lbs. become 10, the 10 lbs. become 20, and so on. Trust me – it's a hard thing to do for me, too. Thank the "full" message delay from the stomach to the brain (among other things), a slow and dangerous 20 minutes or so trip, which is a big design flaw in humans. How can you over-come that problem? Different things work for different people, so here are a few suggestions:

- Decide what you <u>want</u> to weigh. If, for example, you are a 5'6" woman weighing 200 lbs. you know you have a prob-lem. Let's assume that you weighed 125 lbs. in your high school days (or would like to weigh this much, maybe for the first time ever as an adult) and etch that weight into your consciousness. That is the target that you will focus on with the precision and unwavering dedication of a laser beam. You will not get there overnight, or in a month, and maybe not in a year. But you will make progress towards that goal every day, despite unavoidable occasional set-backs. And just like you should not focus on running 26.2 miles at the start of the marathon, but instead focus on a solid first mile, your daily goal is to weigh just a little bit less than you weigh now. Your *numero uno* goal in life for tomorrow: weigh in at 199 lbs. or less. Pencil that number into the scale placemat! Keep it in front of you at every meal (O.K., you may not want to bring it to work or to a restaurant …) and make your food and portion choices accordingly. Keep an eye on everything on your plate and ask yourself if this amount of food will help you lose weight. Will you succeed every single day? No way – you have to anticipate occasional weight swings, re-set your sights, and stay on course. Never give up! To that effect ….

- Start every day with a weigh-in. The truth may hurt, but you don't have to share it with anybody else. **This is crucial – don't omit this absolutely necessary part of your regime.** *Start to worry about your weight when you are 2 or 3 pounds over your normal weight – not 20 or 30!* Make sure you have a good scale, and with "good" I don't necessarily mean "expensive" or even "accurate". All you need is a scale that is consistent: step on it several times in a row and the weight should never vary, or no more than ½-pound maximum. (I prefer a digital scale that only shows ½-lb. increments; no need to micro-worry about ounces, squinting at the display from an angle, etc.)

  Weigh in every morning, and write it down – always. Some nutritional authorities suggest weighing in only once a week (or even once a month), so as not to get discouraged over normal weight fluctuations from one day to the next. Don't believe it. I have seen my weight change from one day to the next by up to 6 lbs. (!), and you know this isn't a "real" gain or loss, but more a factor of hydration, fuel retention, metabolism, bowel movements, physical activities, food choices, timing of meals, etc. Chances are you'll see an adjustment the next day, and you'll get over that "shock" quickly. If, on the other hand, you only weigh in once a week, how would you like to experience one of these freak [temporary] weight gains on weigh-in day – thinking you blew your diet, and not getting a truer picture of your 'real' weight until a week later? You won't be a happy camper for that week, might possibly abandon all plans to ever lose weight again and generally feel miserable. And, assuming you manage to lose weight several days in a row, isn't "immediate rewards" a great feeling, vs. waiting for a whole week?

- **"Happiness is a small, early dinner"** (And sometimes, a *skipped* dinner.) - try it, and see for yourself. Have that small dinner, just big enough to tide you over till breakfast, and early enough in the day before your metabolism goes into hibernation for the night. There's nothing greater than waking up "light", feeling more energetic – and hungry for a healthy (but still reasonably sized) breakfast.

- Having eaten that properly portioned meal as outlined above, **STOP eating after you are done. No seconds. No dessert treats.** No more "just one more taste", especially sweet ones. It could be the start of a cycle of many more "last ones", as each sugar feeding results in an addictive desire to have yet another one. Visualize that scale that you'll step on the next morning. How bad do you want to see 199 lbs. vs. 201 lbs., or 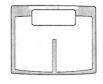 more? Seeing a weight gain can ruin your day, but seeing a weight loss will put a smile on your face, and result in that "I can handle anything that comes my way" attitude. Chances are you'll never win an Olympic gold medal, and I won't either. But if you hit your daily target weight (less than the previous day, or the same if you are in your perfect weight range) you, too, will feel like a champion all day.

Still can't convince yourself to skip that post-dinner treat? O.K., commit to having it – but the next morning prior to your workout. Now you have accomplished TWO things: you have saved those unnecessary calories for the day, and you have given yourself an incentive to get up and have that treat – as a reward for, say, taking a brisk 30 minute walk. Over the years I have fought many battles trying to get out of bed early for some scheduled workout, and what usually wins out is not so much the workout (although I <u>always</u> feel better afterwards, and I <u>always</u> feel cranky if I miss it; eventually one learns), but the fact that I got ready the night before, have all my exercise clothes ready to go – and a pre-workout snack ready and waiting for me. Side benefit: you are more likely to choose a small, <u>healthy</u>, yet still great-tasting snack, since you don't want to see it again during or after your workout, or at the least don't want to feel sluggish during exercising.

- **Before every meal or snack, think first: will this food advance my cause (to reach my target weight safely), or jeopardize my goal?** That extra moment of reminding yourself can be a powerful motivator to "do the right thing", rather than indiscriminatingly eating the wrong foods, or consuming too many calories. **Visualize that scale again.** You have a serious long-term plan, and every small step along the way is important. Ask yourself if the snack you are about to have will really improve the quality of your life beyond the few seconds it will take to consume it, vs. hours of feeling full and guilty. Think of it as a "happiness factor" and, if you are seriously overweight, your life can depend on making those decisions.

- **Get competitive!** We all have a competitive streak in us. How can you channel that to a healthy advantage? Let's assume you have prepared your meals and or snacks for the next day, and it's time to sit down and eat. Look at this snack (and every other one for that day) and *think how much of it you can skip* (save for the next day) and still get a balanced meal and adequate calories. You can't – or shouldn't – starve yourself, but take an honest inventory of what you could do without, then put it away and have your (now reduced) meal. Wow! That should make you feel really good – you are getting control of your food vs. the other way around. And you get to subtract all those calories from that day (and subsequent ones), and you are that much closer to your goal – losing weight one half pound (or more) at a time. Repeat the next day – maybe go for a record low weight? No 'sandbagging' here … like inflating your meal plans so you can cut out more. Use that strategy also in restaurants (which should be avoided as much as possible, due to loss of control of portion sizes and ingredients) and take an inventory of your (most likely oversized) serving. Before you dig in, decide what you can do without and separate it from the rest. You could ask for a to-go container right then and pack it away for the next day. It would be hard (to say nothing of embarrassing) to go back to your to-go container and eat more/all of it!

- **If all else fails** - and un-needed calories are still "calling" you, just walk away from them; physically separate yourself from temptation. Take a walk. Play with your kids. Work on a project. Call a long-winded friend. Wash the car. Ride your stationary bike. Take a shower. Read something really interesting (like another chapter of this book!). Whatever it takes – just don't give in to the temptation to add calories that will truly be "one minute on your lips, forever on your hips". Old, corny advice, but still true. Believe in the power of that 25 minute delay after which your brain will no longer ask for unnecessary calories. Put a timing device to good use: a Timex™ watch works great. So does an egg timer, or an alarm clock – whatever it takes to keep you away from calories for 25 minutes after any meal. And this would also be a great time to turn off the TV or computer, leave the kitchen, and head outside for that brisk walk.

- **More often than not perceived "hunger" is really thirst!** As much as I disagree with drinking large quantities of liquids with meals, it may be the lesser evil if it avoids bingeing on un-needed calories. A glass of cold water, hot fruit tea, or a low-calorie drink like "Fuze Slen-derize® or "Sobe Zero Calories"®, or similar, may be all you need to feel full really quickly – and lose that craving for any more food. Try it as a last resort before giving in to that post-dinner (or anytime else) craving, and see how it goes away after drinking 8-16 oz.

- **Still can't think of anything but food?** Maybe, just maybe, you really didn't eat enough for that last meal or snack. <u>Be honest with yourself.</u> If you truly feel like you need more to eat than planned, just have your next snack sooner. And if that craving hits just before bed time, and you know you didn't eat enough, choose a healthy snack that will be just (barely) big enough to keep you from waking up in the middle of the night with a growling stomach – and raiding the refrigerator (have a drink instead, non-alcoholic and low-cal of course).

- **O.K. – it can (and will) happen: you "sinned"** - and blew your diet. Worse, you know that you blew it and you are overcome by the feeling that, since you sabotaged your weight loss plan already, it doesn't matter anymore and you might as well "pig out". **Stop right there!** You cannot change whatever damage you did already (bulimia is not an option). *But you can stop the damage, and not make things worse.* You can recover from that occasional splurge, that "falling off the wagon". But you have to "get a grip" and not add even worse (too many) calories to already consumed "bad" (too many) calories (even if these calories come from the healthiest sources). <u>Stop right then and there</u> and at least you can take comfort in the fact that you regained control and that "it could have been worse". Make your next meal smaller, or delay it, or cancel it, and before you know it you are back on track. You may not have won that last battle, but doggone it - **you are going to win that war!**

With any and all of the above and other weight loss strategies, you have to be honest with yourself and you have to **want** it to work. If you really prefer to wallow in self-pity and want to prove that no weight-loss/management regime works for you it will be a self-fulfilling prophecy. Pick one or several strategies, as outlined above – but believe in them and want it bad enough to be successful. It can be done – with consistency and long-term determination. Of course if you have serious underlying health issues you will need serious medical help – so check with your doctor first before subscribing to any weight loss plan.

SO WHAT ABOUT GRAINS –
DO WE NEED THEM?

Are grains the "good guys" we can't live without, or the "bad guys" we should avoid?

Nothing is safe anymore; just when we thought it was beyond discussion that (whole) grains are the foundation of good health (just like the food pyramid implies ...), some heretics want to tear it all down - downright sacrilegious. Maybe so, but it would be prudent to examine even the status of sacred cows and see if they deserve to occupy the nutritional moral high ground.

"Grains are the staff of life"
vs.
"The adoption of agriculture was the worst
mistake in human history"

Strong, polarizing opinions I would say, so let's take a better look at them. But first, let's clarify that we are discussing <u>whole</u> grains only, for there is universal agreement that processed, white grains and the resulting grain products are but poor facsimiles of the real, whole thing, and are major contributors to what has been termed "civilization diseases".

The "pro grains" camp can argue convincingly that whole grains have served mankind well for thousands of years, without which whole civilizations might have collapsed, and that they are nutritional powerhouses, loaded with low-glycemic carbs, proteins, some fat, minerals, vitamins, trace elements, fiber, and more. They also made explosive population growth possible by delivering calorie-dense foods in great quantities at fairly steady, predictable rates, and at affordable prices. What's not to like?

"A lot", according to studies of respected scientists. For over **99%** of the time that the genus "homo" existed (think 2 million years!) mankind survived quite nicely without grains. And also existed

96

without infectious disease epidemics, famines, obesity, mass war-fare, and a host of other ills unknown until grains became a staple for humans – only some 10,000 years ago (a mere blip on the evolutionary screen). Also, the greater density of rapidly growing urban centers was not a boon for mankind, but rather laid the foundation for catastrophic endemic diseases, increased stress levels, reduction in food quality in exchange for food quantity, and indirectly for a lot of other societal ills. Merely questioning the supremacy and wholesome goodness of grains appears heretic to many, if not most, modern-day Homo sapiens. Yet it is hard to argue with a successful system that lasted some 2 million years – the hunter-gatherer lifestyle, where animal protein, roots, nuts and seeds, and plant foods were all that was needed to sustain life – <u>healthy</u> life at that. And then there is the incriminating case of some of the most wide-spread food allergies of them all: wheat and soy allergies, compliments of a shift in agriculture to large-scale commercial crop production in depleted soils.

Books have been written about the pros and cons of these vastly different lifestyles, so how are we to think of it? If trained scientific minds cannot agree, how can we decide for ourselves in the trenches? Especially since a convincing argument can be made that after some 10,000 years, humans have adapted pretty well to grains. Or, we've adapted at least to those whole grains grown on small farms practicing crop rotation, in other words prior to wholesale refining coming into widespread use in the late 19th century. There are even theories out that some "newer" blood types (especially "A") have a direct influence on the digestibility of grains – more arguments for the "pro grain" camp. It keeps getting more confusing and more controversial.

So is there an easy solution to the "no grains" vs. "all grains" puzzle? I think so: while the jury is out (and likely to be deadlocked for a long time, if not forever), it would behoove us to remind ourselves to steer clear of the potentially most dangerous diet of all – *the exclusionary diet, no* matter how well intentioned its purpose of eliminating all that's "bad for us" is. Chances are we do not have to tear down the whole house but can just replace a few pieces of rotten timber. What's rotten in our house - all refined-into-oblivion, pasty-white grains and grain products - has to go. All of it. Yes, that includes donuts and other such monstrosities disguising as foods, but also that great-tasting baguette, croissants, Kipferl, Danish, cinnamon buns, 99% of all the "breads" in the supermarket aisle, and white pasta in any shape or size. (Keep in mind that "have to go" is not synonymous with "cannot have ever again". As always, think moderation.)

And while we are at it, we should consider going wheat-free also, since the abundance of wheat allergies is probably a warning sign that maybe we'd be better off without it. Ditto for other gluten-containing grains like rye and barley – we'd probably do well to curtail consumption of these. Just because you don't have full blown celiac disease doesn't mean gluten doesn't cause intestinal problems for you. "Conventional wisdom" tries to convince us that only 1% of the population suffers from celiac disease and cannot digest gluten properly. The implied message is that the vast majority (99%) has no such issues. That seems a bit too convenient: I am not a scientist … but wouldn't it be more plausible that there is a vast gray area of people having sensitivity issues to varying degrees, and that they could be helped by cutting out gluten-containing foods? It would appear that the best approach would be to eliminate gluten-containing foods for several days and see how it affects you. Many people who have tried that approach report a feeling of increased well-being, having more energy, and enjoying better digestion. And as long as you make healthy food choices to make up for that "loss" of a source of calories, and take a daily multi-vitamin/mineral supplement, you shouldn't run the risk of nutritional deficiencies, although you should always consult with your health-care professional when making new lifestyle choices.

"But what about bread – I need bread!" you say? At least that's what some professional cyclists said when the team dietician put them on a gluten-free diet. When, after a few weeks of training and competing they realized that they had fewer abdominal issues and performed better, they didn't miss the traditional fare with an emphasis on white bread and pasta quite so much anymore. Switching to a gluten-free and/or low grain diet is more an issue of behavioral "want" vs. nutritional "need", since staples that have been part of our lives and culture for so long are not easily discarded. Nor, do they have to be. Oriental pasta dishes rely mostly on "rice sticks" (naturally gluten-free), and they end up with some of the tastiest carbo meals available. Then there's <u>gluten-free bread</u>, tasting every bit as good – probably better - as the fare we are used to: "Food for Life"™ puts out excellent brown rice and millet-based breads that will satisfy your bread cravings. And many supermarkets have dedicated shelf space to gluten-free foods, so a lack of variety is quickly becoming a non-issue. Also, be honest with yourself: if the bread you "can't live without" (?) is merely a "delivery system" for the foods you put on / in them, then your problem is not of a nutritional nature, but one of "logistics".

One way to reduce your heavy reliance on gluten-containing grains for carbohydrates is to replace "delivery system" – type breads with gluten-free breads or root vegetables. *Don't laugh until you try it.* Cook up some taro ($1.00 p. lb. vs. $5.00 p. 5oz bag of trendy taro chips, and even a bargain compared to breads), slice it, and then use as a wholesome, minimally processed, natural new "delivery system". Once cooked you can even toast it like bread, and it brings a whole new taste experience to your table. Ditto for other, even less common roots – experiment with boniata root, malanga roots, parsnips, sweet potatoes, beets, etc. How? Easy – just clean thoroughly (some, like taro, have to be peeled), wrap in aluminum foil, add water and/or olive oil, and bake for approx. 45 minutes at 390°F (some more, some less; experiment). And some firm tofu, sliced thin and toasted, makes a great protein-rich "delivery system" too. No, not that ghastly white stuff they sell in most supermarkets, floating in water. Think outside the box and venture into an Oriental supermarket where the variety of sizes, textures, shapes, and tastes of tofu is staggering – and you are likely to find one or more types you'll love. These bread "alternatives" may not work for all the traditional bread uses, but why not experiment, discover new foods, and increase variety at the same time?

But wait – oatmeal has been shown to lower cholesterol! Oh really? How sure can we be that it was the **inclusion** of major quantities of oatmeal and not the **exclusion** of foods it replaced? Maybe the test subjects gave up daily triple egg omelets with bacon and buttered toast to make room for heaping bowls of oatmeal. And if the theory holds true that dietary cholesterol has no impact on blood cholesterol (in healthy people) all bets are off.

Not willing to give up on grains? Go ahead and enjoy them (in moderation), but in <u>whole-grain</u> form. It's neither rocket science nor tremendously time consuming to cook up a batch of organic brown rice, or millet, or quinoa or amaranth, or others. Once cooked, grains can be stored in the refrigerator or freezer for several days or weeks. You may want to experiment though and **eliminate gluten-containing grains for a week or two and see how your system responds.** Feel better than ever? Bingo – you may have found a solution for a problem that you had for your whole life without even knowing about it. Just make sure that <u>any</u> grains in your diet do not become the bigger-than-life foundation in *your* food pyramid (11 servings of a food that until recently – in relative terms – wasn't even on humans' dietary radar screen? I think not. Make the switch to the Food Ark™). And "no grains" is not synonymous with "no carbohydrates". No, these carbs should be replaced with other, plant-based carbs coming from vegetables, fruit, and root vegetables. I believe the no-grain camp has time on its side and the better arguments, but there is no need to apply "zero tolerance" thinking to your diet.

Does it 'work'? Personally I have <u>cut down the use of grains considerably</u> (resulting in athletic improvements), but believe the moderate consumption of them is probably safe, and convenient for everyday realities. An easier question to answer is which are the "good grains" vs. the "bad grains"? Although there are some remnants of benefits left in processed white grains, they would fall squarely into the "avoid at all costs" bad category, while moderate amounts of all gluten-free whole grains (but not necessarily all whole-grain products) can be considered "O.K.". Keep in mind that a host of "civilization diseases" (high blood pressure, diabetes, obesity, high cholesterol, cancers, etc.) were virtually unknown in aboriginal populations worldwide, regardless of the actual diet they ate – and still do in some isolated cases. The Eskimos thrive on a high protein diet of mostly seafood; aboriginals in Australia and Africa rely on "bush meat", grubs, root vegetables, and berries, with fish added whenever possible. The diets of many Asian cultures rely heavily on seafood, other animal proteins, tofu, tempeh, generous servings of vegetables – and, sadly, inferior white rice. And then there is the famous Mediterranean Diet, which supposedly delivers us to the promised land of being able to indulge in real food without gaining weight or increasing cardiovascular risk factors. It's hard to argue with a diet consisting of <u>moderate</u> amounts of animal protein (mostly fish; some lamb and goat meat; some poultry and eggs), <u>moderate</u> dairy products, <u>high consumption</u> of vegetables, fruit and olive oil, and <u>moderate</u> quantities of wine. Notice how the word "moderate" is used frequently to describe this diet. What's not talked about when gushing about the "Mediterranean Diet" (really a diet of the peoples of Crete and southern Italy, but let's not quibble) is that these studies ….

- Looked at dietary patterns that existed in the sixties (!), and ….
- Never made lifestyles a part of the equation (!)

This does not by any means discredit the theories around the Mediterranean Diet, but rather puts the spotlight on the narrow scope of thinking when it comes to nutritional science. For one, the (little) meat these people ate most definitely was not delivered by an 18-wheeler from mega-cattle killing fields several day trips away, and therefore was not chock-a-block full of growth hormones, antibiotics and other drugs. The lamb and goats back in the 60s in those parts of the world (and many other parts) would be considered "pasture-raised & organic" - lean and containing fewer saturated fats, since the animals grew up on native grasses that they found in the (organic) fields surrounding the villages. And you just know that these people were a lot more active then the vast majority of Americans are today, either farming the land, or walking everywhere, climbing, hiking, rowing, and generally performing a lot of manual activities. Given that lifestyle and quality of food, just about any (indigenous) diet would "work" and be of great health benefit to its people. So by all means let's learn from people who live in harmony with the land they occupy, but let's not elevate one diet to near-sainthood levels, without giving other successful diets equal consideration.

O.K., SO YOU DECIDED LIFE IS NOT WORTH LIVING WITHOUT GRAINS

Are there some grains that are better than others? Sure, you could split hairs and look at individual ingredients, and – depending on what appears to be "more important" factors than others (Amino acid profile? Mineral content? Fiber content? Glycemic load?) you could then "rank" the grains, but that would miss the point – again. Looking at the (near-) molecular level of food has not proven to be a successful strategy in the past, so why should it be any different this time? Talk about the total being bigger than the sum of its parts, and keep in mind that new ingredients and functions of basic foods (not to mention inter-connectivity of individual ingredients) are still being discovered, a process that is likely to go on for a long time to come. No, the overriding concern as far as which grain to choose should be "as great a variety as possible" (which does not mean big quantities). Even if grains should turn out to be truly the source of mankind's rapidly declining health, limiting the total quantities eaten, and not putting all your (grain) eggs squarely into the one, say wheat 'basket', would appear to either limit the damage, or provide the greatest benefits. I think the "take home" message should be

- Limit total intake of whole grains and eliminate all processed grains
- Stick with gluten-free grains (brown rice, millet, buckwheat, quinoa, teff, amaranth, corn, sorghum) and consume a wide variety of them – time to discover new foods
- Use organic grains whenever possible

MORE IMPORTANTLY, HOW CAN I FILL THE VOID IN MY DIET WITH REDUCED (OR ELIMINATED) INTAKE OF GRAINS?

For one, your body would thank you profusely if you gave up the most common forms of grains in the American diet altogether: processed white flour products. Sugar-laden cereals in particular manage to make an already bad product even worse (topped off with the colostrum of a different species brings it down several more notches). They are the epitome of "empty calories" regardless of perceived "health claims" jumping off the cereal boxes. Just say no. At the very least find brands that have either no added sweeteners at all (add your own – healthier ones), or very low amounts of "natural" sweeteners. Think "One Ingredient Cereals" like Puffed (Brown) Rice, Puffed Millet, Puffed Corn, and old-fashioned oatmeal (not the instant variety, or sugar-laden ones), or some types of cereals from Nature's Path™, Barbara's™, Erewhon™, etc. Brown rice – based cereals are probably best.

One place to avoid: the supermarket bread aisle. I would estimate that over 90% of what is being sold as "bread" there is directly harmful to your health in the long run. Starting out with denuded white flour again, "improved" by "enrichment", and trailed by a long list of sometimes 30 or more ingredients that our ancestors (even the ones that ate grains) never heard of, and never needed. Preservatives, dough conditioners, fillers, unpronounceable / unrecognizable ingredients, corn syrup or HFCS (high fructose corn syrup), refined sugar, and much more in a product that many still associate with a healthy diet – one that needs only a handful of wholesome ingredients. And don't be fooled by pillowy-soft "Whole Wheat Bread" misnomers that either have only a small portion of whole grains in them, or at best contain 100% of finely ground-into-submission flour from grains grown on mega-industrial lots. No, if you must have bread, stick with the real whole grain kinds: Ezekiel™ is one brand, Adventist™ another, very similar one, and there is Alvarado Bakery™, Mestemacher™ or Feldkamp™ German Bread, or Food for Life™ products, including gluten-free varieties. Their products deserve to be called bread, and if the health arguments won't win you over, the taste will.

How about pasta? All those healthy, happy Italians and carbo-loading marathoners can't be wrong – say it ain't so! Sorry to say, but no matter how you package and market it, most pasta is just the same over-processed white flour product that has a terrible track record when it comes to maintaining human health. Can't live without it? Try buckwheat noodles (usually "whole"), brown rice pasta, "rice sticks", and other 100% whole grain varieties, although that doesn't elevate pasta to health food, in my opinion. Sure, the concentrated energy contained in pasta, delivered to your bloodstream in lightning speed may have some benefits after endurance events, but in most cases the surplus high-glycemic load carbs derived from pasta mostly end up as fat throughout our bodies. Carbo-load (or just satisfy your energy cravings) with low-glycemic sweet potatoes, other roots (taro, boniata, yucca, potatoes, parsnips, rutabagas, beets, carrots, daikons & radishes, celery root, turnips, malanga, arrow, lotus, etc.) instead. And add fresh vegetables and fruit of course.

Still, you insist, what do I eat INSTEAD?

You can't go wrong with upping your intake of healthy servings of vegetables (a variety of cruciferous, green-leafy, red, white, yellow, etc.), root vegetables and fruit, to make up for pasta/bread - calorie losses. Fruit (watch total sugar intake; go for variety in textures and colors again), quality proteins, seeds and nuts (watch caloric intake), tofu, and tempeh should be part of your dietary intake on a regular basis. (No tired tofu jokes please, they haven't been funny since Ronald Reagan was in office. All you have to do to become a believer in those products is try some of the many ways to prepare them in authentic Oriental restaurants, or shop in Oriental supermarkets.) If you think that a reduction of grain intake will affect your diversity of foods, think again: most grain products on American dinner plates are mono-culture, (refined) wheat and corn based, so chances are you are cutting out only one or two (unhealthy) foods. If, instead you are willing to broaden your horizon to include new-for-you vegetables, tofu dishes, root vegetables, and a <u>greater variety</u> of quality protein choices, many of you will end up EXPANDING the diversity of foods consumed, and replace unhealthy, civilization diseases–causing foods with a greater variety of health-protecting foods. Not a bad trade-off I would say. Did you know that many ancient hunter-gatherers had a more varied diet than the typical "Western Diet" of today? They adjusted for seasonally available plant foods (when they were at their nutritional and taste peak), and whatever game animal they could hunt down at any given time (they weren't choosy), or fish they could catch or barter for.

SO WHAT'S THE WORST THAT CAN HAPPEN IF I CONTINUE TO EAT TOO MANY GRAINS?

For one, the more unhealthy <u>processed</u> variety you eat, the more you fail to prepare your body to defend against cancers and other civilization diseases. That's why a little (quality whole grains) goes a long way. Equally important, your first priority may not be to live saintly-healthy but to lose weight. Grains, especially the processed white grains, grown in depleted soils, and containing virtually empty calories only will torpedo your weight loss plans in more ways than one.

- Any surplus energy-dense grain calories will be readily converted to fat.

- Your body may actually crave all the vital nutrients it needs for optimum health, so it may "demand" more nutrient-poor food until all the nutrients are furnished – with a whole lot of empty-calorie baggage to go along. Welcome to the "overfed & under-nourished" vicious cycle. Hard to lose or maintain weight this way. Hard like "impossible".

- Satiety signals often come too late, since hardly any bulk or fiber is left in those depleted grains, so it is easier to over-eat without even noticing.

- Similar to sugar, these processed grains have a high glycemic load, meaning they reach your bloodstream very quickly, cause a "sugar-high", followed by a sugar crash, creating more demand for calories you don't really need. An hour or two after a large meal containing mostly refined grains you are likely to feel like a freight train hit you square-on. Fiber-rich vegetables and fruit, as well as (healthy) fat-containing foods (moderate amounts of gluten-free grains optional) will even out the sugar peaks and valleys and provide a longer feeling of fullness, thereby actually reducing demand and caloric intake.

- The unseen danger of processed foods is even bigger: it's not the damage they can do to the body ("donuts aren't going to kill me"), but what they crowd out of your diet. Every "junk" calorie means another "quality", cancer-fighting calorie <u>less</u> in your system. Or obesity-fighting calorie, diabetes preventing calorie, cardiovascular disease - fighting calorie, and so on. You need all the help you can get just to stay ahead of 21st century stress, pollution, the sleep deficit you keep accumulating, too little exercise, having your defenses up against infectious diseases, and possible other health-threatening factors.

<u>The short list of "good" (gluten-free) grains:</u>

Brown (unpolished) rice, millet, buckwheat, quinoa, teff, amaranth (not technically a grain), corn, sorghum, and possibly "old-fashioned" (not instant) oats (gluten-free status disputed)

For more information about grains and other foods that should be part of your diet refer to the "The Basics" chapter.

THE SWEET TOOTH

SUGAR ...... FRIEND OR FOE ......?

"It is the fuel (carbohydrate) that provides the energy the body needs to function"....

"It is the biggest scourge of mankind"....

"It is an addictive drug"....

"It is your friend during physical exertion and indispensable for maximum athletic performance"....

"It will destroy your teeth, upset your body's mineral balance and is a major cause of obesity"....

And on and on the arguments rage – sugar elicits strong reactions from all corners, so let's separate fact from fiction.

- For one, it is NOT one of the 3 (or 4 or 5 or 6) major food groups. Humans could happily live healthy lives without ever ingesting a single gram of added sugar.

- It is however the fuel your body thrives on – but the human body very efficiently obtains all the glucose it needs from simple and complex carbohydrates, and to a lesser extent from proteins and even fats.

- And even if sugar (glucose) was furnished to the body only via natural foods such as fruit, vegetables, grains, etc. it is still possible to get "too much of a good thing". Fresh fruit may have one of the world's best P.R. agents, but just because a moderate amount of fruit as part of a balanced diet is a very positive thing, too much of a good thing is not wonderful. (Mae West was wrong.)

- As to the relative health benefits of "natural" sweeteners such as honey, maple syrup, brown rice syrup, agave syrup, molasses, brown sugar, turbinado sugar, cane crystals, dehydrated cane juice, etc. vs. the ubiquitous pink, blue or yellow packets of artificial sweeteners, opinions vary widely. Let's just say there are a lot of gray areas. Further confusing the subject is a new breed of non-caloric sweeteners, some more "natural" than others. Think xylitol, sorbitol, stevia, maltose, maltodextrin, erythritol, and more.

The best possible solution: avoid all kinds of added sweeteners, relying on the natural sugar contents of natural foods. Can't do that? I can't either, and admit to a sweet tooth. Blame my upbringing in the pastry capital of the world. Or increased carb cravings due to an intense exercise schedule - it doesn't really matter. Being able to add some sweetness to certain foods and beverages sometimes just plain increases enjoyment of them. And for me at least, it makes healthy green tea palatable, so maybe adding a little "bad" to obtain a lot of "good" is not a bad – occasional – trade-off. Life is not perfect.

Which to choose – artificial sweeteners that **may** cause cancers and digestive problems, or "natural" sugar in its various forms that **will** result in tooth decay and mineral imbalances? Sometimes in life one has to pick the "least bad" options, so here is my take: the pink, yellow and blue packets **may** contain carcinogens – or may not, depending on which expert you want to believe. Real sugar, refined or otherwise, **will** however rot your teeth out slowly, and I would consider losing natural teeth a major factor on the quality of life scale.

But there are better choices out there. The one sweetener that has never caused me (or anybody else as far as I know) any problems whatsoever – even with relatively large quantities - is **stevia**. If it doesn't cause any abdominal distress when consumed right before and during a hard 5K or marathon, it can be trusted to "sit well" in everyday situations too, and there are no known side effects. But it has a flavor of its own that some people find objectionable. Truvia™ is another new calorie-free sweetener – and they largely eliminated that unpleasant-to-some stevia taste. It lists erythritol and rebiana (derived from the stevia plant) as ingredients. And plain erythritol is available online and in some stores, and is also considered free of side effects or abdominal discomfort.

So what other healthy options exist? **Xylitol** appears to be another healthy choice. Safe for diabetics, and actually beneficial for your teeth, this sugar alcohol was originally derived from birch, but now is made from corn cobs also. But it is not calorie-free (it has however approx. 40% fewer calories than decidedly unhealthy regular sugar), and can cause bloating and even diarrhea if consumed in significant quantities, especially if you are not used to consuming it. The only sweeteners (besides stevia and erythritol) that appear to cause no abdominal discomfort seem to be the yellow, pink and blue varieties (also "race-tested", but with difficult-to-ascertain health hazards). The blue type has gotten too much bad press over the years (google "aspartame side effects" and you get 218,000 results, and counting). And why would so many products be advertised as "aspartame-free"? **Drop the blue** – and take your cues from the simple fact that it's already banned outright in some countries.

Helpful hint: if you need 4 packets or more of any sweetener in the (normal-sized) beverage or food of your choice, you are using too much. Try combining, say one yellow or one pink (sans dextrose) with a few drops of stevia, for "turbo-charged" sweetening power. There, you saved 50% of a questionable sugar substitute, since the combined sweetening effect of different artificial sweeteners appears to be greater than simply adding more of the same. (But, don't be mislead by the "zero calorie sweetener" falsehood – they are "cooking the numbers" and most of the pink, yellow & blue varieties contain dextrose, plain old sugar by another name, plus maltodextrin, to the tune of 4-5 calories p. packet.)

Not so quick you say (smugly maybe) – I use only natural sugar (vs. the refined white or pseudo-natural brown sugar), or honey, or brown rice syrup, or agave syrup, or barley malt, etc., and practice good oral hygiene, like brushing my teeth immediately after consuming sugary foods. Sorry, not good enough. For one, too much sugar in your diet will upset your body's mineral balance (especially the magnesium-calcium ratio) that you can't brush away, resulting in poor calcium absorption, something that women in particular can ill afford. For another, brushing immediately after a sugary or acidic snack will do more harm than good, since the tooth enamel has been temporarily softened and can be weakened by immediate brushing. And we are not even scratching the surface of the many other negative health issues associated with sugar such as a suppressed immune system, effect on blood sugar levels, raised insulin levels, weight gain, increased cholesterol levels, over-acidic stomach, headaches, increased blood pressure, leached minerals, and on and on. The common saying in the medical community of **"sugar feeds cancer"** alone should be warning enough to steer clear of this addictive drug, masquerading as food, regardless of type. Using only very small quantities, like a little maple syrup on the occasional (whole grain) pancake breakfast? No need to be fanatical about it – enjoy that 'treat', but don't make it a daily occurrence.

What about all the other sweeteners out there? Chances are they carry warning labels for a good reason. "Excessive consumption may cause diarrhea" is 'code' for 'even normal consumption will make you an unpleasant presence in closed quarters'. Sorry, no free lunch in life when it comes to sugar, so if you can:

- Avoid refined sugar altogether. That seems do-able, and significant health improvements (and weight loss!) tend to be the result. (However, if Tante Hilda baked a traditional cake for your once-every-5-year visits, don't be a jerk and enjoy a piece)

- Use stevia, xylitol, erythritol, truvia™, and if all fails *minimal* quantities of sugar substitutes such as yellow and pink. A little goes a long way, and gradually reducing sweetening agents will wean you away from *excessive* sweet cravings.

- **Skip the blue!**

- "Natural" sugars in the form of honey, brown rice syrup, maple syrup, agave syrup, etc. and too much fruit, especially in the form of juice, are still bad news for your body. At the very least combine sugary foods with foods containing fat, protein and fiber, to slow down the absorption and avoid that sugar "hit" that can send your pancreas into convulsions, figuratively speaking. No orange juice just to quench your thirst, waffles with syrup and sweetened coffee, or a big serving of Sugar Bomb cereal. Wait, did I just describe a typical breakfast in your life? I hope not.

Bottom Line: sugar is a nutritional **'false prophet'** of the worst kind. It promises a quick "hit" of energy combined with a brief feeling of euphoria and immediate satisfaction, and then will desert you when you come crashing down, demand more "hits". It will impact your mineral balance, crowd out healthy calories, pave the road towards addiction and subsequent obesity with all its health hazards, get you on a never-ending guilt trip, and viciously attack your teeth. **Don't. Go. Down. That. Road!**

HERE IS THE MILLION-DOLLAR QUESTION: HOW CAN I KICK MY SWEET CRAVINGS

For one, it's not easy, but several strategies work. And all successful strategies have one thing in common: you have to believe in them, and stick with them. Some people can cure their sweet tooth "cold turkey" from one day to the next and never miss it again, while with others (the truly addicted) it's more like A.A. – they have to resist temptation on a daily basis for the rest of their lives (it tends to get easier).

To begin with you would do well to take stock of the extent of your sugar addiction and ask yourself as a reasonable person if it is worth it. Is any piece of candy or chocolate or cake or cookie or soft drink or other source of empty sweet calories worth all the

misery? Before you say 'YES' emphatically ("life without chocolate isn't worth living") consider the hazards:

- Obesity, with associated loss of self-esteem, confidence,
  reduced earning power, social stigma, embarrassment, etc.
  – and I don't even include health issues at this point.
  Chances are this "only happens to other people", right?
  Read on - obesity can lead to ...

- Diabetes and all its complications. It's not just about
  adjusting your diet (there go all the sweet things in your
  life). Instead, think fatigue. Think impaired vision. Think
  skin breakdown. Think joint disease. Think wheel chair.
  Think amputated limbs. Think organ failure. *Think about
  it.*

- Cardiovascular disease: yup, The Big One – M.I., aka
  "heart attack". Most people get smart after their first one.
  But not all. You may want to give some thought to getting
  smart BEFORE a heart attack. By-pass surgery is no fun
  whatsoever. It's not routine, it's not "business as usual" for
  a long time again ("never" for some business), and despite
  the best drugs money can buy (yours, or your insurance
  company's) it is painful – and remains like that for a long
  time.

- A shortened lifespan: "no sweat" you say, assuming you
  are young and the concept of living beyond 50 is horrify-
  ing anyway. I am cool with that – but **you may not be**
  when you leave your loved ones to fend for themselves
  and you don't even see your children graduate (or they'll
  push you there in a wheelchair). And besides financial
  riches, **chances are excellent that your children will
  also inherit a vastly reduced life span from you.** Vastly,
  like *decades* shorter. That's right, research has shown that
  the offspring (and their offspring!) of people who gorged
  themselves for relatively short periods of time in their
  lives (less than a year) tend to die at a much younger age

than the offspring of healthy-weight people. How much do you love your children?

Has any of this gotten your attention? I hope so – but I am not optimistic. Addictions tend not to be logical. But at least you know you <u>should</u> change your way – and don't know how. Try any or all of the strategies below, but you have to be honest with yourself and sincerely **want** to kick the sweet-tooth habit that you know can ruin your quality of life – or your life. **Commit to it!**

- An Australian study group conducted an interesting **experiment**: sugar-addicted people would be served their favorite sweet fix, but were not allowed to touch it. So there sat that chocolate cake (or think of your favorite 'downfall') and people just stared at it. They monitored heartbeat, sweat rate, salivation, etc. and – no surprise there – they all increased measurably. After a few minutes (longer for some people than others) a funny thing happened – all readings went down or even returned to normal. The cravings had weakened or disappeared, and they could walk away from their 'treat' without touching it (!). This approach has promise, and you have nothing to lose by trying it, so you may want to give it a shot sometimes. At the very least you could get that sweet you can't live without (?) served up nicely (have a container ready to pack it up again ….) and think it over for a good long time, considering the consequences. How about putting it away for a later time – like a pre-workout snack, or as part of an otherwise healthy meal. **Visualize that scale** that you will step on the next morning. Not fleetingly, but think it through. How would it make you feel if you saw a weight loss the next morning, even by just ½ lb? 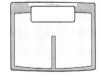 Wouldn't that signal a positive first step that could literally "make your day"? Isn't 24 hours of relative happiness worth a moment of denial, or at least delayed gratification? Wouldn't "just saying no" to that sweet fixture in your life feel empowering? Seeing smaller numbers at the weigh-in every morning should be The Number One Priority in your life – because it can save your life in the long term, and make you feel better (vastly better!) in the short term. Don't let go of that vision, no matter what.

- **Don't go for that post-meal sweet treat.** No, not even that "one small taste". You are an addict, remember, and your body cannot be trusted. It will ask for just another, and another, and before you know it you have added serious excess 'garbage' calories to your diet. *You are dangerously overloading the pleasure pathways* in your brain and will have to consume more and more to get the same amount of pleasure. It's a nasty downward spiral, feeding on itself, with every sugar "hit" making it that much harder to resist the next one. Making things worse is that hormonal disruptions brought on by too much sugar consumption may send more (false) hunger signals to your brain! If laboratory test animals are any indication you may even turn down foods other than sugar and/or fat-laden empty-calorie snacks, just so you can get to your 'drug'. Instead, make good use of a timing device and WAIT until time's up (at least 25 minutes) before you even think about anything else – by then your brain will have received the "all full" signal from your stomach – **listen to it!** You will feel full, maybe even uncomfortably so. Don't add to your misery! Go for a brisk walk instead. Immerse yourself in a project. Call a friend or a relative. Get on your stationery bike. Leave the kitchen – or the house. You could even call it "flee the kitchen". Or brush your teeth and call it over for the day, after dinner (the most dangerous time to give in to your sweet tooth), since you should feel reluctant to eat anything after brushing your teeth. And don't sit in front of the TV – to see junk food commercials or have a bowl of M & Ms handy.

- **Commit to having a healthy snack prior to having anything sweet.** Maybe a few slices of cucumber (mucho alkaline)? Or the appropriately named sweet potato (no added sweetener needed). Or a few salty nuts, veggie chips, wasabi peas – anything that will take that sweet craving right out of your mouth. Not in the mood for any of these – well, at least you have established that it's not hunger driving your cravings, so don't add unneeded calories – of any kind. You could also give in to that sweet craving – but with a beverage, which not only can satisfy your sweet cravings but also tends to give you that full feeling. Licorice tea anyone? Not your cup of tea? How about a non-caloric yet sweet drink? This could be plain water (always your best choice), or fruit tea with stevia, diluted fruit juice (don't go overboard), soup, or decaf coffee. There are even some reasonably healthy ready-made beverages out there, like "Fuze Slenderize"™ or "Sobe"™ Zero-Calorie fruit-flavored drinks. Having any of these "pre-sweet" snacks (salty is better!) or beverages will most likely kill the desire to have that (additional) sweet snack, especially if you wait for at least 25 minutes after your "good" snack.

- <u>Cut down</u> **on the sweeteners you use.** Can't quit cold turkey? I would think this would be near-impossible for many. So cut back in stages, to a point, where sweet things mean less and less to you. For starters replace real sugar (all kinds) with stevia, xylitol, truvia™ or, if necessary, small amounts of the yellow and pink (look for varieties without dextrose). This isn't perfect, but it's a step in the right direction. Can't live without "the real thing"? Actually you'll live a lot longer without it. Try living without it, and you may make a surprising discovery: stay away from sugary beverages or sugar-containing foods long enough, and the alternatively-sweetened versions will actually taste better! Also, give this a try: prepare a beverage that you usually sweeten and have a few sips without <u>any</u> sweetener. Tastes awful, right? But you may notice that you'll actually taste the flavor of the beverage. O.K. – this is not going down, so add a small amount of sweetener (say, ¼ of what you would usually use). Huge improvement, no? Not any-where good enough, but take a few more sips. Enough of that? O.K. – add another ¼ of the usual amount of sweet-ener. At this point your cup of tea (or other beverage) has already "shrunk" by a good amount, so the total amount of sweetener you put in until now (still only ½ of the usual!) should make this cup of tea palatable. Finish it – congrat-ulations, you have just cut your sweetener consumption in half! If you don't succeed at first …. try again, maybe only reducing your sweetener intake by one quarter, then aim for additional reductions during subsequent days. Use this concept with every sweetened food, and you'll discover how the real taste of any food will come to the forefront.

- **Do you know how much sweetener you consume?** Start keeping track of it. As an exercise, keep all the yel-low or pink envelopes you use in a day (or jot down every spoonful of sugar, or xylitol, etc.) and tally them up. Then commit to using 10% or 25% or 50% less of it every day for a week or so. Keep downsizing your sweetener "ration" until you have made a significant reduction in consumption. Surprise: after doing this long enough, less sweetened foods and beverages will taste just fine, maybe even better, since your taste buds get used to real food fla-vor again which hasn't been overpowered by gobs of sweeteners. Bonus: you may sleep better too.

- **Visualize.** Humor me on this. Visualize all the healthy foods and beverages you put into your system, unadulter-ated by empty calories, and only in the quantities you need. Visualize how your body will thrive on it, heal itself, and rid itself of a substance (sugar) every bit as addictive (and damaging to your health) as nicotine or caffeine. Visualize putting only premium fuel into your body – the only one you'll ever have. It can be a powerful and empowering feeling. Try it for one single meal and see, then repeat it if you like what you 'see'.

- **Get angry!** It's not you against that donut, or sugary soft drink, or candy bar. They are just means to an end for the manufacturers of these products – to profit off you and your health. You should be angry at them, for they have engineered their offerings to get you addicted, and in the process have deprived you of your body's natural food instincts. They have managed to "brain wash" your sensation of taste to react only to hyper-sweet things, and weakened your normal desire for complex carbohydrates in the form of vegetables, fruit, root vegetables and whole grains to the point where it is not strong enough to resist their empty calorie designer "foods". They messed you up and you are not going to take it anymore - **you want your life back!** If you don't reclaim it, you will throw good money after bad – to the healthcare industry to treat your high blood pressure, high cholesterol, diabetes, etc. Don't let them get away with it!

IS THIS A GOOD TIME TO TALK ABOUT CHOCOLATE?

To some people it is ALWAYS a good time to talk about chocolate, since they consider it one of the major food groups, at least in their personalized food pyramid. It too has found a slick P.R. agent that transformed this food f.k.a. junk food into health food. Strangely it is adopted as such (health food) most often by people who still refer to people eating *real*, healthy food as "health nuts". Go figure. Anyway, chocolate is a good example of how a mildly healthy raw ingredient (100% cocoa, non-alkalized) is overwhelmed by the negative health problems associated with the added ingredients to make it taste – and sell – better: sugar, dairy fat, and various fillers, preservatives and such. By the time you buy that designer chocolate bar for "health reasons" (wink, wink) all that unhealthy baggage has long ago overpowered the few, feeble good-for-you properties. Why does this remind me of Playboy readers who buy the magazine only to read the good articles? (Yeah, right.)

No, if you really, really want to consume chocolate for health purposes buy 100% chocolate from Ghirardelli™ or 100% cocoa powder (non alkalized) and either eat (or drink) it 'as is'. This is hard to swallow … so add reasonably healthy sweeteners, or the "least unhealthy sweeteners", which will still be better for you than what the chocolate manufacturers use in their products (they try to make a tidy profit – think cheap ingredients). Try these treats that should take care of your chocolate cravings: Laura Scudder's™ Natural Peanut Butter on top of a piece of 100% Ghirardelli™ chocolate and (optionally) sweetened with stevia and possibly some erythritol or xylitol. Or 100% cocoa powder stirred into hot almond (or rice) milk & water, sweetened with same "least unhealthy sweeteners" of your choice. Now you could call those moderate quantities of chocolate "healthy".

A WORD ABOUT FUEL DURING COMPETITION OR HARD TRAINING

There is one occasion when the use of sugary foods is difficult to eliminate – during and immediately after athletic competitions. Even there, too much sugar can lead to intestinal problems during long endurance events, so at the very least pick low sugar options such as "Mojo"™ bars by Clif™ (typically 9g of sugar vs. 20 or more per bar), "Think Thin"™ protein bars (sugar alcohols, but -0-g sugars, and still 20g of carbs), or at the very least bars with no added REFINED sugar. Clif™ and Odwalla™ bars would be good candidates, as would be any of the "Organic Food Bars"™ (gluten-free, alkaline forming and great tasting), and all Envirokidz™ bars — also gluten-free. Best of the bunch: **Lärabar™** - sometimes only TWO all natural ingredients and usually no more than FIVE – they are the least processed bars, are gluten-free, kosher and vegan, and have no added sugars whatsoever. Not surprisingly they also taste great. Mind you, these are processed foods, not health foods, but during races or as an occasional snack they beat most, if not all, the other snack options. If you see "sugar" or "high fructose corn syrup" or the ingredient list, let your competitor get sick on them and avoid them as snack options anytime.

Your better strategy may still be to plan ahead and pack some snacks made from "real food". Some athletes have good results munching on cooked **potatoes** or **sweet potatoes**, and I know cooked **taro** slices work great. Need something more mainstream? Pitted **dates** or old fashioned **peanut butter sandwiches** (no-sugar-added jelly optional) sit well, and if you add a dash of salt, chances are you'll never need another salt tablet in your life. (I wouldn't know what one looks like, and have never dehydrated in my life, including at the 113 degree Ironman China in '09.) And bananas are truly man's (and woman's) best friend during competition.

What about gels? As much as I hate to admit it, they serve a purpose at endurance events, especially during the last leg of a
triathlon or ultra run, since the overriding concern is how fuel
will be tolerated by the stomach. Gel brands like Hammer™ or
Carb Boom™ or GU™ seem to have the least amount of simple
sugars, yet are still high in carbs, and generally sit well. Ditto for
Cytomax™ Performance Drink — it "sits" rock solid during
high-intensity runs. Just don't use gels exclusively for events lasting longer than 2-3 hours, with the possible exception of **Accel**
gel. **Hammer Perpetuem**™ is the fuel of choice then, or GNC's
"Amplified Endurance Booster"™. And keep in mind that
adding "real" food like aforementioned PB sandwiches or
bananas will extend your meaningful "life" on a long run by
avoiding or delaying sugar overload which can result in abdominal distress with all its ugly consequences.

Happy racing, and once your race is over and you've had your
protein-carb recovery drink, get off the sugar roller coaster.
Remember, sugar is **not** your friend.

SO WHAT ARE THE BIGGEST FACTORS FOR HEALTH AND LONGEVITY?

Actually they are not food items at all. Overall you can improve your health and increase longevity best by quitting smoking, using seat belts, not drinking alcohol or use other addictive drugs. But I am convinced that the single biggest *dietary improvement* you can make to your health – and for weight reduction - is eliminating all refined sugars and greatly reducing your intake of all other sugars. When I finally realized that sugar was not a benign race fuel befitting my athletic lifestyle, something unexpected happened, despite being race-lean already: I lost weight, without even trying! I felt better too, had more energy, and my quality of sleep improved. Like so many changes in my habits on the road to the "perfect diet" (it's a journey, not a destination), I tried something positive, with no iron-clad intention of sticking to it forevermore, then liked the results so much I never went back to the "bad old ways". You may want to take a similar approach, since it is mentally a lot easier to make healthy changes on a "trial basis", and then decide if the results are worth sticking to your new ways. But trust me on this one – you will notice an improvement if you **cut out the sugar.**

VEGETARIANISM

True vegetarians do not consume any meats or animal products, including honey, milk, eggs, etc. This group of people is sometimes referred to as "Vegans". Since I could never quite subscribe to the logic of calling somebody who consumes eggs and dairy products a "vegetarian" – neither food grows in soil or on trees after all – I will mean *"vegan"* whenever I discuss a *vegetarian* lifestyle. If animal-based foods are added to a purely vegetarian diet this would be called lacto-ovo, or pesco-, or semi-, or any number of "other" vegetarian. That includes, but is not limited to "sometimes vegetarians", fruitarians, flexitarians, and many others. One can carry this to extremes, like only consuming organic plants that died a natural death (O.K., I exaggerate on the last one – I think).

The benefits of most of these diets and lifestyles are real, and well documented: lower mortality rates from all major diseases, lower weight, lower blood pressure, lower cholesterol readings, fewer cancers, less diabetes, and a better sense of well-being due to fewer intestinal problems, a less acidic body, a more active metabolism, and reduced stress, and less aggressive behavior patterns. And let's not forget the much smaller impact on the environment, much more efficient utilization of available food sources, and the positive vibes for "doing the right thing", by eating plants, not animals that have been raised in <u>unfathomable cruelty</u>.

So why aren't we all vegetarians? Leaving alone tradition and taste preferences and many people's insistence on having a piece of meat or fish on their plates, why wouldn't more people choose a vegetarian lifestyle?

For starters, early humans were "survivatarians" out of necessity – it was a fight for survival, **all** the time. They wouldn't have survived for millions of years being picky about their food choices – it was tons of wooly mammoth meat at one time, followed by tree bark at other times – and anything in between. They had to get their life-sustaining protein from the first available, most abundant sources – other animals, and carbohydrates from plants and fruit they could find. Any which way you slice it, humans are omnivores, and they survived for millions of years that way – long before grains were cultivated or widely available. That didn't happen until the relatively recent 10,000 years or so. Two million years is a long time to get used to a certain diet, and it may appear unwise to try to fix something that's far from broken. What IS broken however is how the system of providing quality animal protein for human consumption has resulted in the deterioration of the final product that ends up on our plates.

Let's consider beef. It's not necessarily that beef is "evil" in and by itself, but rather what has happened to it over the decades. Next time you are in the supermarket compare the nutritional data of regular beef to venison or buffalo meat, both largely unchanged for hundreds, if not thousands, of years. The difference in fat and protein content, cholesterol and sodium is huge – and this doesn't even reflect the vastly inferior diets today's cattle are fed, with added growth hormones, antibiotics, and other drugs. It is these unseen "ingredients" resulting in unseen "obesogens" that are largely responsible for a final product that is far less wholesome than it was even a few generations ago. The picture for commercially-raised poultry vs. pasture-raised poultry, or farm-raised seafood vs. wild-caught is equally bad, or worse. Without going into great detail (which could be a whole new book), suffice it to say that "evil" animal protein used to be much healthier than it is today. This development has resulted in, among other things, an increase in the popularity of vegetarian diets, when the answer should really be making sure to get adequate amounts of **high quality** animal proteins instead of the wholesale <u>elimination</u> of all animal proteins. Strict vegetarians have to scramble to consume adequate amounts of quality protein, which is the first step towards the most dangerous diet of all – **the exclusionary diet**. Most vegetarians don't fall into that trap, but many people do, without being aware of it, driven by the desire to eliminate all "bad-for-you" foods, sometimes skipping meals or making poor choices resulting in unbalanced meals.

There are other problems with strict vegetarian diets:

- Nutritional deficiencies: yes, I know, a properly planned vegetarian diet can be balanced, healthy, and provide all the nutrients known to be necessary for human health. There you have it – but the devil is in the details. Apart from needing to have the prerequisite (extensive!) knowledge to be a successful vegetarian and painstaking execution of meal plans, getting "all the nutrients *known* [at this time] to be necessary for human health" may not all be available in non-animal sources. We don't know, since we know better than to believe that nutritional science has discovered all there is to know about human nutrition. We do know however, that vitamin B12 and iron are usually too low in vegetarian diets to avoid deficiencies, and have to be taken in the form of supplements. Deficiencies for zinc, calcium, vitamin D, and vitamin B6 are also more common among strict vegetarians. How many other nutrients are missing in a strict vegetarian diet? We just don't know yet, and we may never fully understand the interaction among all nutrients.

- Protein requirements: yes, it is possible to satisfy the body's protein needs with a strictly vegetarian diet. In order to do this successfully different types of protein sources have to be combined in order to obtain the 8 essential amino acids the human body cannot synthesize. Some vegetarians side-step that requirement and use a variety of protein powders (soy, rice, pea, potato, hemp, etc.) to satisfy their requirements, which is neither very tasty nor wholesome-natural. More typically vegetarians combine **legumes with (whole) grains** or **legumes with nuts** or **legumes with seeds** to offset one group low in certain amino acids with another group high in those amino acids. One drawback of this concept is the fact that large amounts of foods have to be consumed just to satisfy protein requirements, coming with lots of fiber, fat, and calorie "baggage" which may not leave enough room for other important foods, like fresh vegetables and fruits for example, and possibly some essential fatty acids. The latest research indicates that this tedious combining of 'complimentary' proteins doesn't have to happen at every meal, but can take place over the entire day, like having legumes (and other foods) for lunch, and whole grains (or nuts or seeds) and other foods for dinner. I don't buy it – and you shouldn't either, and it's not because the science is flawed (it probably isn't). But even **if** the "all day combining" theory is sound, it makes meal planning even more daunting, since in the "real (hectic) world" many people can't remember in the evening what they had for lunch, much less breakfast. If you take your chances with combining vegetarian protein sources, your safest bet would be to have each and every meal balanced.

- Insufficient knowledge: anybody who embarks on a strictly vegetarian diet without doing extensive research will fail in their goal of improving their diet and health. Just yanking the meat off the dinner plate and not making any other changes to one's diet (including adding supplements) is a dangerous concept. Imbalanced nutrient intake, possibly compounded by choosing refined sugar and flour (or white rice) products over whole grains, consuming too much sugar, and not consuming a wide <u>variety</u> of vegetables, fruits, legumes, nuts, and seeds, etc. can add up to a ticking time bomb, since sometimes deficiencies do not manifest themselves until the damage is done.

- Poor absorption: <u>as humans age, foods are less easily absorbed</u>, and legumes – a cornerstone of vegetarian diets - are hard to digest even under the best of circumstances, as are nuts and seeds to some extent. This means that normal loss of muscle mass may accelerate, making a bad situation worse, so as you get older you may want to re-evaluate your lifestyle choices.

Don't think for a moment that I am hostile to the concept of vegetarianism: I was a happy strict vegetarian ("vegan") for several years and loved it. But when my health and athletic performance started to decline slightly and nutritional deficiencies were the probable culprit I opted to add fish, and eventually organic eggs and small amounts of venison and buffalo meat to my diet as a dietary **"insurance policy"**. My health improved, as did my athletic "career" when I stopped being a strict vegetarian, which would seem to confirm that I made the right decision. But as always, just because a little (quality animal protein) is good, a lot is definitely not better, and a "mostly vegetarian" diet would appear to be the safe and healthy way to go.

Your best strategy: substitute the occasional meat dish with vegetarian fare. If 90% of the US population adopted healthier vegetarian diet choices just a few times a week, the positive impact on the health of the people <u>and</u> the environment would be far greater than if 20% adopted a strict vegetarian lifestyle. Plus the former is attainable; the latter may be neither attainable nor desirable.

STAYING HEALTHY LONGER

I don't want to read about old age and all that" successful aging" garbage. I intend to be successful at <u>staying young!</u>

Well, this is what this chapter is all about! Read on to see how you get 'there'.

For starters, think back at a time when you were sick – really, miserably sick. Say, food poisoning, or a bad injury, or a kidney stone, or a painful meeting with your dentist. Chances are you were so miserable you might have said something like "I'll do *anything* to feel good again – **anything***!*" That's a situation you want to avoid in old age – when pain like this could be <u>chronic</u> - let me make this clear, "chronic" like "forever" and "chronic" like "won't go away". Also, keep in mind that the *"I'll do anything!"* sentiment is heard and understood, and taken advantage of by the healthcare system. So not only does it hurt, things may never be "like they used to be", and what limited improvements you can achieve *will cost you dearly*. Maybe doing the right things <u>NOW</u> to avoid finding yourself in such a tight spot <u>later</u> wouldn't be such a bad idea. Feeling good, a general absence of pain and avoiding "adult failure to thrive" is what it's all about. Assuming you don't plan to "live fast and die young" (you wouldn't read this book then) it doesn't matter how old you think you'll get, but *you want to maintain the best quality of life for as long as possible.*

What does that have to do with a book about losing weight? **Everything.** Not only do obese people have shorter life spans, more importantly their *quality of life* is impacted severely. Old age symptoms will set in earlier, and ill health is practically a <u>given</u> if good dietary habits are not followed and proper weight is not maintained. "No worries – I won't live that long"? Nice try, but no matter how long (or short!) you live, you don't want to live in pain and discomfort for years before your untimely demise, no matter when that is, so it wouldn't hurt to get prepared for what's coming your way. Books have been written on the subject of "successful aging", which is surprising considering how little the subject has been studied, but a few facts are known. Here's a short, and by no means complete, list of what we can expect as the years add up:

1.   Muscle tissue declines with age, with a corresponding increase in fat, especially around the internal organs. That means just maintaining your weight will be a tough battle, and even if successful, chances are there's less muscle and more fat on your body.

2.   Your BMR (basal metabolic rate) declines with age, resulting in fewer calories burned for the same activities. Approx. 7 per day (fewer calories for every year) for men, 10 for women (life isn't fair).

3.   Since calorie requirements generally are less as we get older, eating nutrient-rich foods becomes even more important. So instead of indulging in "discretionary calories" (a nice term for junk food, empty calories, decadent treats, alcohol and such) more often, we can afford poor nutritional choices less often in our later years.

4.   Bone density goes down! That's especially worrisome for elderly women who have to make sure their calcium, vitamin "D", magnesium and protein intakes are adequate.

5.   Oral health declines, resulting in reduced chewing (masticating) capabilities, avoiding certain foods, and less salivary flow when taking prescription drugs (which has a big negative effect on dental health). To make matters worse, many older people develop a sweet tooth (or never lost it in the first place) leading to dental caries. The net result of all or some of these factors will be even faster deterioration of dental health and malnutrition symptoms.

6. Protein absorption decreases with age. This is a big one! At a time when the aging body naturally loses muscle mass, less quality protein is absorbed to stop the decline.

7. Rates of constipation increase with age – up to 60% of some age groups use laxatives, making a bad situation worse.

8. Malnutrition is a major factor, maybe **the** major factor that can cause cancer. And you can reverse that last sentence: cancers and their resulting treatment often lead to malnutrition.

9. Compounding all these factors is the fact that older adults are less likely to make dietary changes, at a time when such changes (to healthier diets) may be critical.

10. Alzheimer's, one of the most dreaded diseases, typically strikes older people – it is the 6th leading cause of death for the over-60 age group.

If this isn't enough bad news already, there's more. In no particular order here's a short list of additional health issues that are far too common among the elderly: anorexia of aging, dehydration, high blood pressure, obesity, cardiovascular disease, diabetes mellitus, renal disease (reduced kidney function), COPD (chronic obstructive pulmonary disease).

So is there **any** good news about getting older? Yes there is, and I am not talking about wisdom, maturity, happiness and such. The good news is that all of the above conditions or changes are not a "given" and can be influenced greatly by lifestyle choices we make, sooner rather than later. Let's re-visit the points above and look at the details:

1. Muscle mass declines with age, but this decline can be slowed tremendously – think **half the loss**, which adds

up to having a lot more functional strength as we grow older. Even untrained older people – in their 90-ies - can **add** muscle mass and **reverse** muscle loss! There you have it – resistance training, truly <u>the closest thing to the "fountain of youth"</u>. Yup, that's right. Pumping iron isn't just for body builders in their prime anymore; the older set needs this type of exercise even more. Of course the best results will be achieved if there is a solid base of proper weight, cardiovascular fitness, and a healthy diet. And don't worry about eye-popping bench presses, super-sets, and hundreds of push-ups. A well-rounded workout program, including resistance & cardiovascular training, core-strength exercises, stretching, balancing, warm-up and warm-down that will leave you invigorated rather than exhausted is all that's needed. Get clearance from your healthcare professional, then have a personal trainer in a fitness center show you the ropes, and you are on your way to feeling 10 to 20 years younger than what your birth certificate says. <u>Visualize that – 10 to 20 years younger!</u> This is not a myth! And chances are you'll meet new friends in the process, and find a support group. What's not to like about that?

2.   To avoid weight gain, caloric intake has to be reduced. Better yet (much better!) burn more calories to make up for this age-related reduced need for calories. That means as we get older we should exercise **more**, not less. I'd consider this good news. With the time restraints of a full-time job and children to care for gone, replace some of these saved hours with active time. Now's your chance to hone your golf game, improve in tennis, or get faster in the pool. Even tending to your garden or taking long walks instead of sitting in front of the tube will keep you burning the same amount of calories – or more – as you always have. You may even see improvements in retirement in "hard core" sports such as competitive running, cycling, swimming, triathlons, weight lifting, etc.

3.   O.K., so the "discretionary calories" should go (most of them, anyway), but is that really such a hard thing to do? By now you know what ice cream and pastries taste like (usually not as good as they look), don't have to 'discover' new junk foods anymore ('been there, done that'), and have less tolerance – and hopefully desire - for alcohol. Instead, challenge your experienced taste buds with new exotic dishes (no, they don't have to be super-spicy, and won't cause ulcers) that are minimally prepared and lower in calories. Most <u>authentic</u> Oriental-Cuisine restaurants offer healthier fare at lower prices, so go ahead and explore.

4.   Osteoporosis is not a given for older women! If you like sardines and canned salmon (<u>with</u> the bones), drink calcium-fortified beverages (there are better choices than milk), eat non-fat yoghurt (if you can't live without dairy products), and enjoy the outdoors to get moderate sun exposure you can greatly reduce your chances of dangerous mineral losses. Weight-bearing exercises (walking, running, resistance training), which have numerous other health benefits as well, are key. And you should probably consider adding a multi vitamin / mineral supplement **and** additional calcium-magnesium-vitamin D to your daily diet.

5.   Declining oral health – now there's a great reason to practice good dental hygiene (yes that includes flossing) and see your friendly dentist at least twice a year. You want to enjoy all your favorite (healthy) foods for as long as you can, so eliminating or greatly reducing your intake of sugar in all its forms (especially the white refined type) becomes more critical. It seems like a fair trade-off – less sugar now, so we can enjoy all other foods much longer.

6.   What to do about poor protein absorption? Eating more, especially poor quality proteins or those that

come with heavy nutritional "baggage" (saturated fat, added fat, cholesterol, obesogens, etc.) is obviously not the answer. The emphasis should be on **quality protein**: a pasture-raised chicken egg most days would be a good start, as would several weekly servings of wild-caught fish (including canned), occasional small servings of venison, buffalo meat or grass-fed, pasture-raised beef, tempeh, tofu, legumes with nuts, or seeds or whole grains, etc. Another way to "cheat" and get more quality protein into your system can be achieved by consuming the occasional (dairy-free, low sugar) protein shake, or adding protein powders to your tea or coffee. This also eliminates other, far less healthful artificial creamers or dairy products. And if you are not doing this already, make sure you consume some raw vegetables or fruit and <u>enzyme supplements</u> to every meal for improved absorption. Thorough chewing will also release more nutrients from your food.

7. Constipation isn't just inconvenient - it can poison your body and make it a fertile ground for cancers to develop. The solution could be as easy as drinking a lot of water or other "good" fluids, consuming more vegetables and fruit, and <u>adding 1-3 tablespoons of ground flaxseeds to your diet.</u> Add a little exercise and you should never have to resort to artificial or "natural" laxatives, all of which have their side effects, not to mention that your body can become dependent on them. Avoid them at all costs, unless they are physician-prescribed and you are under medical supervision, in which case you better check with your doctor first.

8. Wouldn't it be nice if you could reduce your chance to get cancer by anywhere from 25 – 80%, depending on the type of cancer? You can, and the "miracle drug" is no drug at all, but a healthy diet consisting of mainly plant foods (organic preferred), quality protein, legumes, nuts, seeds, herbs, plenty of liquids (filtered

water is best), combined with moderate (at a minimum) amounts of physical activity. Also remember that _"sugar feeds cancer"_ and that obesity is a major underlying condition for cancers to develop and thrive. "Super-Foods" said to deny cancers a foothold in your body include beans, berries, cruciferous vegetables, dark green leafy vegetables, flaxseeds (ground), garlic, onions, grapes and grape juice (skip the wine or drink in moderation; **avoid** resveratrol!), tofu & tempeh, tomatoes, whole grains – and probably many other natural foods. Seen any of these foods at your local fast-food restaurant lately? Think about that.

9. Just because you have eaten red beans and rice with ham hocks and sausage all your life doesn't mean your life will have no meaning without these foods. Just skip the ham hocks and sausage and "bury" some tofu or tempeh in there, change to brown rice and it's "all the taste without the baggage" and, with higher nutritional value dialed in. Ditto for white rice and refried beans with flour tortillas – switch to plain beans without added grease or bacon, corn tortillas, brown rice, and voilà – your dinner now deserves to be called healthy. Use that kind of thinking with other ethnic dishes or just plain old family favorites – and of course venture out and find new, healthy favorites too.

10. Is there a cure for Alzheimer's yet? Not to my knowledge (but they are working on it), and even the causes for it are not well understood. However, you may be able to reduce the odds of getting it greatly. Healthy diets such as the Mediterranean Diet, with a high intake of fresh vegetables and fruit, moderate consumption of animal proteins (mainly fish), healthy fats (olive oil), etc. may offer some protection, although it appears too soon to make a definite statement. Ditto for turmeric, which has many proven and yet-to-be-confirmed health benefits, and may be a factor in the defense against

Alzheimer's disease. Until "they" figure it out you can't go wrong trying just such a diet (or Asian diet, and other healthy diets) rich in anti-oxidants (vitamins C, E, selenium, carotenoids), essential fatty acids and B vitamins. And it always seems to come down to an active lifestyle: regular exercise is linked to a lower risk of Alzheimer's disease. Bonus: exercise may also cut your risk of contracting age-related macular degeneration by up to 70%.

Bottom Line: like it or not, **old age will happen**, and what's good for us NOW will reap even more benefits LATER. More and more, scientific findings suggest that <u>declines typically associated with aging are more a result of **lack of activity**</u>, as well as other poor lifestyle choices. It was not too long ago that people in their sixties were considered old (sometimes meaning "frail"), yet there are men in their seventies now who can run sub-3 hour marathons (no, not me – yet: I'll let you know when I get there). In any event - think **"use it or lose it"**.

SHOULD YOU GO BEYOND AN ACTIVE LIFESTYLE?

Will you benefit from taking the next step – becoming athletic? Why should you invest immeasurably more effort to get there, when all the (sweat) investments tend to yield more, yet diminishing (health) returns? Well for one, you do get healthier as you get leaner and more athletic, by virtue of getting more exercise, following a well-planned workout routine, and increasing the intensity of your workouts. That's why "more is better" in this case. (When you train at world-class, ultra-competitive levels, additional health benefits can sometimes be outweighed by health detractors – not a worry for the vast majority of mere mortals.)

For another, shifting the focus from "can't eat this, shouldn't eat that" to an athletic goal that is reachable, makes the weight-loss effort secondary. Trust me – if you go from brisk walker to finishing near the top of your age group in a half-marathon, love handles will not be on your worry list. Losing excess weight, then, becomes a secondary goal and you find that meeting the race goal is somewhat more under your control.

How do you get there? Just like you have to crawl before you can walk, and walk before you can run, you have to become "healthy" (get into an acceptable weight range) before you can get "fit" (adding regular physical activity, of both cardio and resistance-type, and don't forget core strength), before you can work on becoming "athletic" (reaching your potential). And to avoid turning this healthy progression into something that can result in negative health effects, check with your healthcare professional before embarking on any strenuous exercise program.

Once you have been cleared to pursue athletic activities start increasing your workouts *gradually*. The biggest mistake newcomers and experienced athletes alike make, is "doing too much too soon", followed closely by not taking the occasional breather - like a weekly rest day or two - or by not including "easy" weeks every 4-6 weeks. Whenever you increase frequency, duration or intensity of your chosen workout(s), do so slowly, over a long period of time, and never all at once. In other words you can go from running 20 miles a week to 22 miles a week – then stay there for another week or two before going to 23 or 24 miles. "Consolidate" those gains before you increase your mileage further. And you do not want to increase your "quality" miles (speed work, tempo runs, races, etc.) relative to your total mileage at the same time. Ditto for jumping from running 3 times a week to running 5 or 6 times a week – you don't want to "go there". Doing so will increase your chances of an injury from "slight" to "it's just a matter of time". Sadly, you cannot trust your instincts on this since muscles and the cardiovascular system respond quickly to training stimuli while bones, joints, connective tissue, ligaments, fascia, etc. take years of slowly increasing loads to become stronger. However, it is that positive feedback from your muscles and increased cardio output that lulls you into a false sense of progress and security. And, because other, slow-developing body capabilities don't jump up and yell "stop – enough already", but quietly do what they are supposed to do, until they cannot handle the workload anymore and break.

So by all means, pick an athletic goal that will keep you motivated, but going from a sedentary lifestyle to becoming a decent marathon runner in 6 months is not a practical target. Sure, you might be able to *finish* a marathon, but that, in and by itself, does not catapult you onto the athletic plateau. You will be much better off if you work on reaching certain "milestones" first, like becoming a proficient 5K runner, building up to 10K distance events, and eventually a half-marathon. This progression can and should take years, and these "stepping stones" are worthy sub-goals in their own right. Who knows, you may decide that you'd rather excel at say, 10K races, than put in all those long, boring miles to become a mediocre marathon runner – and get injured. Or you may add bicycling to the mix and compete successfully in duathlons. And you may take the next step and become a multisport athlete and do triathlons, adventure races, or pursue goals in other sports.

WHY YOU CAN'T EXERCISE

Let me count the ways …. there can be many reasons, some legit, some just excuses.

For starters, you are exercising already - a lot actually, whether you want to admit to it or not. Unless you are bedridden or comatose you burn a lot of calories just doing everyday chores, like walking around, driving to work, carrying groceries, playing with your children, eating, even just sitting in front of the computer or reading this book – or sleeping for that matter, along with hundreds of other daily activities. And no, it's not insignificant. The calories you burn in a week doing what most people would consider just normal activities of being alive (called non-exercise activity thermo-genesis) are more than you would burn running 35 miles a week. Pretty n.e.a.t, eh? But you are not off the hook – there are huge benefits to be gained by performing additional, **planned** exercises (not surprisingly called exercise activity thermo-genesis) – and it doesn't have to be 35 miles of running.

So why are so many people dead fast opposed to anything that hints at sweat-inducing physical activities, despite the overwhelming evidence of their health benefits? And what are the reasons most often cited for staying on the couch?

Let's look at legit reasons why you feel you can't exercise (or have no desire to) first, aka "The Short List".

- You have an existing medical condition, or are morbidly obese, which prevents you from doing anything strenuous. My heart goes out to you, and I hope you see your doctor or a specialist for advice. Even these special population groups can usually participate in medically supervised activities, so discuss this subject with you doctor.

- You are stuck on the space station, and the weightless treadmill and Zero-Gravity ExerCycle are broken.

137

- You are in a maximum-security jail in solitary confinement.

None of these reasons apply to you? Then I cannot think of any other reasons why you cannot find minimal time for meaningful physical activity, so let's move on to the reasons that "qualify" as excuses for some people, and I'll try my best to *disqualify* them.

- The number one reason given for not exercising: *"I don't have time to exercise"*. Chances are you knew that. Long hours in the office, 2 jobs to keep a roof over your head, long commutes, being a single parent, etc. are all tough hurdles to clear, but they are not insurmountable. Remember the old saying that **"He/she who cannot find time for exercise will have to find time for disease"**. Take your pick.

  For one, there is the financial toll any illness takes on you, above and beyond the physical pain you have to endure. So just looking at it from a medical expense point of view, whatever time you invest into being healthy and physically active will pay big dividends down the line in reduced medical bills. And of course <u>you will be of no use to your family if you are laid up in bed</u> or the hospital, but be a burden on them instead. So, carving out that small amount of time for yourself to work out is not selfish, but quite the opposite. Sadly, "spare time" will not jump up and demand your attention and make you go out and do something active, fun, and at least mildly strenuous. There are always other projects around the house, chores, things to do with the kids, vehicles to wash, lawns to mow, dinner to cook, and so on. Even the sock drawer needs organizing more than your body needs physical activity, or so it seems. *"I know I should exercise"* is a sentiment one can push ahead of reality for a very, very long time. You are in a "no exercise" rut, admit it.

O.K., if you know you <u>should</u> exercise, but never get around to it, then maybe it's time you tried a different approach. Rather than waiting for that spare time to jump up at you, with running shoes in tow, **just plan for it - NOW!** The best way I have found to defeat the defeatist "I have no time to exercise" attitude: make it your **first priority.** Just get up and do it, preferably first thing in the morning, then let all the other important (and not so important) matters battle it out for the remaining time.

Set the alarm clock 30-60 minutes earlier than usual (how about doing this right now?!). I'll let you in on a great secret: getting up ½- hour or 1 hour later doesn't make getting out of bed any easier. So, set that alarm, have all your workout gear and a small snack ready before you go to bed, and when the alarm goes off don't question it, don't think about it, don't think about reasons why you shouldn't get up – just think of that pre-workout snack calling you and **get out of bed.** Put the alarm out of reach (but within earshot) so you have to get up to turn it off, if that's what it takes. Think that you **will** feel better after the workout than before you get started, no matter when you get up – I can guarantee that. If you get your workout done in the morning you don't have to worry about missing it in the evening, sometimes for reasons beyond your control. Bonus: you will feel better all day!

O.K., so you "fall" out of bed, **determined**. Worry about all the reasons why you should sleep in later, and once you've splashed some cold water in your face, gotten dressed for the occasion, and you are up and awake you will feel way too committed to go back to bed. Congratulations, you have just taken the first step towards a healthier you! What about all that sleep that your body needs? A sleep deficit is a bad thing to keep pushing ahead of you, you say. I agree, but sometimes the (little) extra time is better spent walking or running or cycling or swimming or working out in the gym rather than fulfilling your sleep quota - especially in light of the fact that Americans spend an average of 3-5 hours a day in front of the TV! And maybe 2-3 hours a day online! Just think of the shape you could be in if you converted just part of this sedentary time into meaningful exercise! Easier said than done? I know – I have been active for over 20 years, and for a long time it seemed like it would never get easier – but it did, eventually. For a habit to become ingrained you have to stick with it for at least six weeks, so find an activity (better yet, *several* activities) you like (or at least some that you don't hate) and stick with it. Making it a social 'thing' is a great help, because you know your buddies are out there waiting for you to run or bike or swim with, or you'll make new friends at the gym and you want to be part of that support group.

A word of caution: you can't – or shouldn't - go from zero to a-mile-a-minute overnight, so pace yourself. Otherwise, you'll either burn out or injure yourself. Schedule 3-5 mornings for (easy at first) workouts, until it becomes a habit. Skip E.R. or The Late Show, cut back on your facebook time, prepare for the next morning's workout, get to bed earlier, set that alarm, and don't question it. You owe it to yourself and your loved ones to give this an honest try for 6 weeks. Before long you should get some positive feedback from your body, telling you how much better it feels, how much more energy you have (a great paradox, that you have to invest energy to get more energy back), and you should start to see the weight, or inches – or both come off.

Follow the same pattern for <u>after-work</u> physical activities: **plan for it**, bring your gear and some (healthy) snacks and water with you to the office and go straight to the gym, or the track, or the pool, or wherever else you are planning to go. I have learned the hard way that going home first, then packing up to go to the gym simply does not work. You come home and you feel beat! Or you see projects. Or you answer the phone or e-mails. The kids are all over you. Time flies, and by the time you have psyched yourself up to head to where you were planning to go, it is too late, or the momentum is lost, and you stay put. I did this even though the Y where I worked out was only 1 mile away. Don't go down that road – this is important: **you must have everything you need for your evening workout with you and go straight to wherever you work out**. Still not convinced that you'll have the time? Think of the man who may have the most stressful job in the world – the President of the United States. Think of Barack Obama what you like, but he is a true role model when it comes to working out (as is his wife), and **always** finds time to stay in shape and healthy. So did his predecessor, George Bush, for that matter, and he too was a role model on that front, if that example appeals to you more. The problem is not the time, but the lack of **planning** for that time. Knowing this, in and by itself, should feel empower-ing. Another way to look at it is by thinking back how you managed (miraculously) to "find" time in the past, for a new hobby which intrigued you, a friend who needed you, you started to work on the deck you had been dreaming about for so long, a new motorcycle which was calling you from the garage, your girlfriend who wanted company to go dress shopping (exciting for ladies only …), or some other reason that 'forced' you to find time. You found time back THEN, and you can PLAN to find time for a health-ier you NOW. **Plan for it!**

- *"I am not athletic, don't have a bike, and certainly am not fit enough to run."* So what's wrong with taking long power walks? It's a no-skills-required healthy activity most everyone can do, with due apologies to the handicapped. And speaking of the handicapped: if you are not, think how many wheelchair-bound men and women would trade all their worldly belongings if only they could walk.

That alone should be motivation enough to go out there and enjoy the activity, just "because you can". Go as slow or as fast as is appropriate for you, and always consult with your doctor if you have not exercised in a few years, or recently had health issues. But get moving, and slowly increase distance or speed or the frequency of your workouts. Walking is still too strenuous or "off limits"? Try water-based exercises – they are probably the best non-impact way to get started, and classes can be found in most Ys or health clubs; they are some of the best-attended classes. Coming to a pool near you soon: underwater treadmills, the ultimate non-impact walking (or running) exercise machine, with benefits ranging from rehabilitation to challenging workouts. If you have access to a gym or a treadmill or own some other exercise equipment, great. If not, just keep walking, maybe with occasional jogs, and keep it fun, yet challenging. Buy that stop watch, record your workouts, and <u>keep track of improvements.</u>

Here's another secret: **The Power of "C"**: the body thrives on it, results **will** come with it, and you **will** feel better and you **will** be healthier with it. It is the ….. "C" word – **CONSISTENCY**. Every workout counts, even if the scale may not show it after one workout. Neither will the mirror. But with lots of "C" in your new lifestyle, results are inevitable. I like to think of health and fitness as a telephone book, with each thin page presenting a workout. That one page is too thin to measure, but just look at the complete residential section of a phone book of any major metropolitan area. If your goal is improved health, with enough consistency your "phone book" will be several hundred pages thick and you will reap the best returns for your (exercise) investments.

If you go beyond that, and "fitness" is your goal, you have to add a lot more pages, and your "phone book" will grow in size. Go for "athletic" and your efforts will show slightly diminishing returns (more work for less gains), yet you will still increase the size of your "phone book" tremendously, until it looks like the New York City phone book (which may be a CD now, but you get the idea). The message there is that **improved health can be achieved with relatively little investment in sweat and time**: no need to be able to run marathons before breakfast, ride a double century, kayak the length of the Mississippi, or swim the English Channel. You may be able to get there one day, but it will take a lot of hard work – a lot more than "just" reaping the health benefits of a relatively modest workout plan. Reach for the easy-to-pick low-hanging fruit of good health first. Take-home message: the more you put into it, the more you'll get out of it, but a little goes a long way.

- *"The equipment needed, or health club membership fees are too expensive"*. Again, think about walking, which only requires good shoes to start with. If you can and want to progress beyond that, consider the money spent on an active lifestyle as the best investment in yourself you can possibly make - literally, by how much you will save in medical expenses, and figuratively, by the improved quality of life you will enjoy. Plus your life may depend on it! Don't wait to get smart until after your first (or second?) heart by-pass surgery. **Get smart NOW and never meet that friendly surgeon in the O.R. - but play racquetball with her instead!**

"Running for your life" can take on a whole different meaning. Adult-onset diabetes is not a "normal" part of aging – you can control your destiny in that regard. Consider this: **50-80% of some cancers in the US are due to lifestyle factors (!!!),** and physical activity could well be the single most important risk-reducing action you can take. Whoever could capture those kinds of cancer risk-reducing properties in a pill would be rich beyond imagination, yet when all that's required are some lifestyle modifications, people lose interest. Don't become a statistic! Medical bills are one of the major reasons for personal bankruptcies, sadly even for people who have health insurance. Don't become a profit center for a hospital! Any major disease like cancer (or bypass surgery, or diabetes, or a number of other "civilization diseases") will be expensive, and painful, and life-altering, much more so than a benign change in diet and exercise habits. The cost of treating chronic illnesses linked to obesity is estimated to be $168 billion dollars a year in this country! That's a staggering amount, but is dwarfed by the cost of medical bills and lost productivity due to cardiovascular disease – a whopping $400 billion dollars a year! That's money that is not available for R&D, the education system, repairing and improving the decaying infrastructure, or any number of other productive causes.

- *"I live in a high-crime neighborhood and walking or running around the block is out of the question."* Sadly I cannot solve the crime problems in many neighborhoods, and I wouldn't hold my breath for the government to do so either. But maybe walking with a friend or a group of friends can make walking or running a safe proposition. And keep in mind that most criminal perpetrators are sound asleep by 5:00AM. Also, think "safety in numbers." Who knows, if you can organize enough like-minded people to walk or jog in your neighborhood maybe **you** can outnumber **them** – or get the local police department to notice and swing into action. Can you get to a safe area where other joggers or walkers meet (mall-walking anyone?), or go to a health club? Some Ys offer lower monthly fees for the financially less fortunate, so you may want to look into that. Can you get some minimal exercise at or near your workplace, either after hours or during lunch? At the very least you should have opportunities for meaningful physical activities during the weekend.

- *"I am embarrassed by the way I look and don't want to be seen at a gym or on the jogging trail"*. Obviously you haven't been to a gym lately. There are lots of overweight and even obese people there who have refused to be self-conscious to the point of not participating in healthy activities. Why not join them and have a ready-made support group? And trust me: everybody at the gym is too focused on getting their own workouts done, and will not be inclined to watch other members sweat. Or you could just walk longer-than-usual wherever, whenever you walk, whether that's outdoors or in a shopping mall.

- *"I am too old."* Older than 90 years? Modified resistance-type workouts under medical supervision have resulted in strength gains for 80 and 90-years olds, improved their functional strength, and have given them greater independence. Gus, one of the regular "active older adults" at the Y I use is 85 years old, so don't feel limited by your age, ever. Regardless of age, if you have not been physically active for a while, check with your doctor first as to what type of exercise, intensity, duration and frequency are appropriate for you. And you might have read success stories about older runners who didn't start to run until they were 50, or 60 or 70, and then went on to run Boston. Or people 50 pounds overweight – or 100! – who lost all their excess weight and became runners. "Miracles" like this don't happen overnight, and there's nothing quick and easy about it, but given enough determination, perseverance, and a healthy serving of the "C" factor (Consistency), anything is possible.

- *"I hate to exercise"* .... *"I cannot stick to an exercise program"* .... *"I get bored"* ..... *etc*. These excuses have one common denominator: you have not found the right activity or the right environment yet – one that you could enjoy. But how many have you tried? Or rather how few? In my opinion, *in order to stick to any exercise program the effort has to be measurable, and/or rewarding, and/or social, and/or show results.* Sweating all alone at home with a workout video may work for some, but the boredom factor is hard to overcome for most. Ditto for cycling nowhere in front of the TV. And rowing machines, stationary bikes, in-home tread-mills, Nordic trainers and such are clogging up the nation's attics and garages.

I have found that the exercise habits that "stick" are the ones where you commit yourself to **go there.** Yes, leave the comfort cocoon of your home and at a set day and time plan on an "away from home" activity. At home you will <u>always</u> find other things to do, or get distracted. Save the money you could spend on a home gym that you can use "at any time" because the time to use it will soon become "later" or "tomorrow" or "after I finish this pro-ject". Before you know it, that workout machine you spent your hard-earned money on becomes an indispensable clothes rack.

Instead, get up and get out of the house. Driving to a health club at a certain day and time of the week, prefer-ably in a group setting, will make it a lot easier to form a habit you can keep. I have contended for years that the hardest part of my resistance workouts was walking down the steps to the basement, where the weight room was. Another way to make a boring workout routine interest-ing is by getting competitive. Instead of mindlessly watching MASH reruns on TV while cycling, or walking the same 1-mile loop over and over again, see how long it takes you to complete a certain workout. A stop watch can be your best friend and best (and cheapest) coach. Take note of the elapsed time, then repeat later during the week or next week, and see if you can "beat your time". Same with the bike: see how many calories you can burn in 20 or 30 or 60 minutes (or how far you can go) or however long your routine is, then try to go further in the same amount of time next time. Get imaginative with repetitive work-outs and/or alternate activities. Tell yourself that "on Monday I'll walk, a day or two later I'll swim, a day or two later I'll spin, then I'll try aqua-jogging". I lucked into triathlons, consisting of 3 sports that challenge all parts of your body and, due to the variety, keep any individual sport from getting boring. All you have to do is look for activities that push your buttons - you can alternate jogging, kick-boxing, weights and yoga, for example, or get into racquetball and Pilates, or any number of other activities. Think *measurable, and/or rewarding, and/or social, and/or prone to show results.*

- ***"I have exercised in the past and didn't see any results"***. For one, keep in mind that "you get out of it what you put into it". Even though walking the dog every morning for 20 minutes is better than watching soaps, it will not melt fat away and build awesome muscles. 30-minutes a day, 3-5 times a week, plus weight resistance and core workouts 2-3 days a week is the gold standard. Sound intimidating? Relax - you can't (and shouldn't) get there in a week, but rather build up slowly. As you increase the time you perform meaningful physical activity (and/or duration and/or intensity, but never all at once) you will feel better and become motivated to stick with whatever you are doing – and do more, until you find the amount of exercise that feels just right for you. You **will** see and feel results with the magic ingredient – CONSISTENCY.

- ***"Last time I exercised I was sore for days."*** O.K. – it happens to Olympic-level athletes and newcomers alike: the "too much – too soon" syndrome. That's no reason to quit; just try again with less intensity or less duration next time, and allow your body to recover and adapt. And never go into a workout program thinking "I was on the track team in high school, surely I can run a 5K next weekend" – when those days were 20, 10, or even just 5 years away, and you haven't laced up running shoes since then. YOU may remember, but your BODY has forgotten a long time ago.

- *"Who will take care of my baby?"* Well, the Y daycare center maybe. Or a friend. Or a spouse. Or maybe you pack the little'un in a baby stroller and see how many "solo" runners you can pass. I'll never forget the dedicated young mom who swam in the lane next to me while her little girl was sound asleep in a baby chair at the side of the pool. If the baby fussed, mom was never more than a few yards away, and she kept active despite what would appear to be an insurmountable problem.

- Here's one most people will not readily admit to: *"I hate to sweat – it is so undignified."* Not as undignified as being wheeled into the O.R. for by-pass surgery dressed in a gown that's flapping open in the back. Come on, this is the 21st century, showers have been around a few hundred years, and there are plenty of active role models among movie stars, socialites, the hyper rich, and royalty. I bet even the Queen of England worked up a good sweat "in her day" horseback riding, or running after her Welsh corgis.

- *"I just don't have the energy to work out".* I feel your pain – no, really. I'll share a discovery I made a long time ago; call it an exercise paradox. Whenever I felt too tired to keep my appointment with the weight room, I would always (like, 100%) feel energized, upbeat, and much better after the workout. And you can experience this paradox yourself, regardless of the type of workout you do. Do it often enough and long enough (say, six weeks or more) and you'll be hooked.

- *"I am too stressed out at work and at home to work out".* Considering that exercise is an excellent stress reducer, you just deprive yourself of a potential cure! One of the body's natural responses to stress is to store more fat, compliments of hormonal imbalances. Therefore the answer is not "less physical activity" but "more", or at least "regular" amounts of time spent being active.

- And finally, what may be the real reason why you don't want to get active: *I don't like to change, and adding exercise to my daily routine would require too many changes in my lifestyle.* You may want to examine if your current way of doing things isn't what got you into trouble in the first place, so maybe it's high time you tried something different. Doing the same thing over and over again (bad diet habits, lack of exercise, not enough sleep, poor lifestyle choices, etc.) and expecting different results is a bit of wishful thinking, no? If whatever you are doing isn't working, why wouldn't you try a new approach? **Now** would be a good time: go for a brisk walk, or set that alarm an hour earlier tomorrow, and work up a good appetite for breakfast. **Plan it – now.** Think of the alternative – how much more your lifestyle would change if one of the preventable civilization diseases put you in the hospital for an extended period of time

In conclusion: there are many "excuses", real or imagined, the most common of which I tried to address, and all of them can be overcome. What you have to do to be successful with a workout program is have a true desire, **make a plan that you can live with**, and execute it. You have to make that switch from "I know I should" or "one of these days I will" to

"I will get up earlier tomorrow morning".

"And I will have all my gear, food and water ready, and **I will do it no matter what.**" *Planning takes no time at all* – you can do it during your commute or your lunch hour, or instead of watching TV. *Preparing for each workout takes minimal time* – how long can it take to get workout clothes and shoes ready, a water bottle and maybe a small snack? When <u>you</u> are ready to commit, it <u>will</u> happen, and the best time to start is not Jan. 1, after a significant birthday, or when your doctor scares you into it. Get smart **before** your first heart attack!

The best time to start is <u>now</u>.

(STILL) POPULAR MYTHS – EXPLODED!

MYTH: "HEALTHY FOODS DON'T TASTE ALL THAT GOOD": Oh, really? This would imply that the cuisines of France, Italy, Greece or Austria (to name just a few) of, say 2-3 generations ago, induced gag reflexes in those poor people who didn't have tasty (?) freeze-dried foods, frozen entrees, and assembly-line baked goods delivered to the restaurant by trucks, or breads baked many miles away in a factory. How did they survive, much less enjoy their meals, without veggies from farms the size of Rhode Island, using trainloads of chemicals in their depleted soils? And without eggs that didn't come off a conveyor belt, laid by c.c. chicken that were fed the cheapest feed packed with a veritable drug cocktail? What, no plastic-wrapped cuts of meat coming from a plant hundreds, or thousands of miles away and containing growth hormones and antibiotics ? Can you imagine life without vacuum-packed snacks with 20, 30 or more ingredients? Life without fast food outlets at every corner? <u>Must have been a drab world.</u>

Still, something strange happened. Tourists from all over the world discovered those "plain" foods, raved about them and eventually created such a demand that ethnic restaurants from these and many other countries sprang up all over the world, supermarkets started carrying their products, and cook books featuring these and other ethnic cuisines became bestsellers. Maybe it's because many of these dishes were prepared using local produce and meats, minimally processed, and served in normal portions. Foods that didn't need ingredient lists and "heart healthy" claims yet were better for our health. Foods that didn't have expiration dates in the distant future. And, most importantly, dishes prepared from those foods that tasted delicious. Bottom Line: new (and definitely not improved) processed foods laden with cheap fats, sugars, sodium and a long list of un-needed and/or un-pronounceable ingredients will never measure up to "real" foods, neither in taste nor healthfulness.

MYTH: "IT'S NOT MY FAULT – I HAVE THE FAT GENE": you may be right – there really is such a gene ("FTO", and there are probably other genes and mechanisms at play, all part of a still poorly understood concept) that can predispose you to pack on extra pounds. The good news: we are talking 1.2-3 kilos here (2.6 – 6.6 lbs.), so in no way, shape or form does genetic disposition account for the other 20, 50 or more pounds that you may carry around with you. Sorry, there goes *that* excuse.

More good news: many people have this gene and are slim and trim. Their secret? Discipline at the dinner table and *physical activity*, which not only burns extra calories but also reduces the effectiveness of the gene. Burn more than 900 additional calories a day and you may be able to 'checkmate' this nasty gene altogether. So genes are not all powerful, life-controlling factors against which we are powerless. Quite the opposite is true – we can alter some genetic traits with appropriate lifestyle choices! Even if the genes themselves don't change, genetic markers (methylations) can change – or inhibit – some genes, via reversible chemical reactions. Epigenetic mechanisms that regulate genes can be influenced towards "bad" or "good" effects, and these epigenetic changes can become hereditary! Smoking, for example, can change the activity of some 300 genes (!), and you know these won't be *good* changes.

On the other hand, adopting healthy lifestyle choices can *positively* affect the activities of 500 genes. These changes (for better or worse) can occur within months! Epigenetic changes can be blamed for the obesity of baby girls born to mothers who ate excessively early in life (and obese boys of men who did the same). However, such changes can also be decidedly positive such as when diet & lifestyle factors can reduce the chances of contracting certain cancers, or when expecting parents embark on a healthy, active lifestyle, with special emphasis on sound nutrition to improve the chances of having healthy children. Genetic and epigenetic research gets messy and über-scientific quickly, and I do not claim to understand it all, but the good that comes out of all this research is that our social environment and lifestyle choices can, to an extent, override our genetic fate. Maybe Hippocrates grasped that concept when he opined "Let food be thy medicine and medicine be thy food".

MYTH: "EATING HEALTHY IS EXPENSIVE": *it doesn't have to be.* Sure, if you replace **all** the things you currently eat and drink with organic products, chances are you'll spend a fortune. But just switching to organic everything (as healthy as that would be) wouldn't really change your diet much, would it? Organic cookies, anyone? And since your current eating habits have gotten you into the trouble you are in right now, not making a *meaningful* change will not get you any different results as far as your (excess) weight is concerned. In order to do that, chances are you need to

1. Eat less in general (and spread your calories out over 4-6 meals / snacks)
2. Eat better quality foods
3. Eliminate poor value-for-money junk foods

   1. Eat less in general: let's assume that you bought this book because you want to shed unwanted pounds. It could well be that you added extra pounds over time by over-eating by a significant amount. So if you consumed 20% too many calories in the past (which only kept your fat cells happy) just by cutting out those extra 20% PLUS another 10% (until your weight has returned to normal), that translates roughly into buying 30% less food!

   2. Eat better quality foods: You can buy a lot of organic products for that 30% you just saved. And the higher quality food will be more nutrient-dense than its conventionally grown counterpart, so you don't have to eat 1-1/2 apples to get 1 apple's worth of quality nutrients. BTW, organic apples often cost the same (and some-

times less) than the conventionally grown variety (shop around), and you avoid the pesticides too. Same with red meat, which should be eaten sparingly anyway, yet 'hogs' way too much space on our collective dinner plates. <u>In order to get the same amount of protein that is contained in a piece of beef of a given size</u> (and which comes with much more saturated fat, cholesterol, and a toxic combination of drug and hormone residues) <u>you get away with eating a much smaller piece of venison or buffalo meat.</u> Hint: ground venison meat can be found at reasonable prices in the freezer section of many supermarkets.

On a budget and can't afford fresh wild-caught salmon? Switch to canned salmon at a fraction of the cost. True, this is not the 'gourmet' option, and you may not want to serve it 'as-is' on your dinner plate when your mother-in-law comes for a visit, but it makes great salmon salad or – spread, and it is usually wild-caught, while most supermarket or (expensive) restaurant salmon never ventured beyond fish ponds, and may have survived (barely) on a sub-standard diet in filthy water. Check out great deals on canned mackerel, sardines, and herring too (all quality protein sources from abundant wild-caught fish), not to mention a wide variety of canned (and fresh) seafood in Oriental supermarkets. Include more inexpensive quality calories in your diet: legumes (beans, lentils, chickpeas, peas, peanuts, etc.) – always a great value for your money; <u>root vegetables</u> - packed with vitamins & minerals, delicious, satisfying, and healthy, low-fat carbohydrate sources (and talk about under-valued, and therefore inexpensive); brown rice; single-ingredient cereals if you can't live without them, like puffed rice, corn or millet (add your own, healthier sweeteners and sweet spices); frozen vegetables and fruit, etc.

3. Eliminate poor value-for-quality junk foods: take a closer look where some of your current food dollar is going and you'll notice that you get little in nutritional return for some foods. Soft drinks are a prime example: refined sugar–only calories (the worst kind) or no calo-

ries at all in the case of diet drinks. What you do get however is a cocktail of mineral-depleting liquids (calcium for one – think osteoporosis), enamel-depleting phosphoric and citric acids, and fizz that may result in retaining water. It's a similar picture for corn and potato chips (too much cheap fat), candy bars (refined sugars and fats), Mega-Bucks lattes (not exactly junk food, but all the calories come from sugar or dairy), most processed foods (cheap flavor enhancers raise the price and reduce quality), candy and chewing gums (addictive, regardless of sweetener used), ready-made sauces or toppings, and many other items.

How about fresh vegetables and fruit, which can be relatively expensive? (This, btw, compliments of our skewed food supply system that subsidizes cheap-to-grow crops to fuel the fast-food industry – and *cars*, yet only gives lip service to the importance of healthy plant food.) Buy seasonal: don't worry about getting **all** the fruits or veggies during any given week – you can get enough variety buying produce that is in season, plentiful, at its nutritional peak and usually a lot cheaper than during other times of the year. Or take advantage of sales, and freeze what you cannot consume within a few days. And some of the best produce deals can be found in the freezer aisle. Picked and processed at their peak (they are also the cheapest then) they retain most, if not all of the nutritional value they had when fresh. Buying like that also avoids bingeing on strawberries when they are in season, only to make do without for the rest of the year. Add frozen strawberries, or blueberries, or cherries (pitted – does life get any better?), or other frozen fruit (organic whenever possible) to fruit teas, cereals, or use them as ice cubes to chill your (non-alcoholic) beverages. This way, your body gets a steady supply of some of the healthiest foods available without breaking the bank, and your body will love the consistency and variety.

Don't have time to chop veggies? Go for those mixed vegetables in the freezer section of your supermarket, steam them, add some (healthy) Mayo (I am partial to Nayo™ or Vegenaise™) and seasonings after they have cooled down, and that bland veggie side dish becomes addictive. Call it "Austrian Gemüsemayonnaise" and you might just confuse your children enough that they'll love it – and eat their veggies in the process. Make sure peas are in there or add canned chickpeas (legumes; buy low-sodium variety), sprinkle in a few nuts or seeds, serve with a slice of tofu or tempeh (gluten-free bread optional), and voilà – you now have a complete and balanced meal, protein, carbs, fiber, and all.

And then there is always the lowly baked potato. Great nutritional value by itself, wholesome, virtually unprocessed, and begging to be topped with healthy things, like chives or other herbs, olive oil or barbecue sauce, nutritional yeast, olives, tomatoes, garlic, etc., but without the deal-killers (butter, sour cream, cheese, and such). Add tofu and nuts or seeds and you'll have a complete meal in no time, at a bargain price.

Bottom Line: be imaginative, expand your culinary horizons (think ethnic cuisines), and experiment with inexpensive yet nutritious foods. Chances are you'll end up with **more** variety, not less, and get better nutritional value for your food $ to boot.

MYTH: *"FREE* FOOD IS ALSO FREE OF CALORIES": of course we all know better, but sure don't act like we do. Take the "free" snacks in your office or plant for example: those donuts or that slice of birthday cake, or a co-worker's party leftovers usually don't last long in most company kitchens. Yet, most people still have all of the lunch they brought to work, or still go out for lunch, or still have the same size dinner, as they would have had without all those "free" calories. Not surprisingly these calories make quick friends with your existing fat cells and settle in for good.

How to deal with it? "Just say no" should work in most circumstances, since most of the time nobody forces food on you anyway (no, that's not the donuts in the kitchen calling you). Chances are you can avoid those diet-busting birthday cakes at work also (blame a recent root canal?), or at the very least have a polite, small piece only. And whenever you cannot avoid "free food" (a potluck Thanksgiving lunch at work would be an 'honorable' example), just call it your meal, and skip or reduce your next meal accordingly.

MYTH: "A CALORIE IS A CALORIE IS A CALORIE ..."
Not so – <u>not all calories are created equal</u>. You know – or should know already – that one gram of one food can contain 4 calories (proteins, carbohydrates) or 7 calories (alcohol) or 9 calories (fat), but did you know that processing all foods you consume is calorie-burning work for your body? That "thermo-genetic effect" is different for each type, and fat requires the least amount of "work" to digest. Calories from carbohydrate use up more energy than fat calories (and complex, low glycemic foods more than refined carbs), and protein takes the most energy. Think of it as a calorie 'rebate': if you were to replace 100% of your fat in any given meal with the exact same caloric content in the form of protein you'd end up with a reduced "net" intake of calories, once processing is subtracted. So why wouldn't we eliminate fats altogether and replace them with quality low-fat or non-fat protein? Don't go there! Apart from the human body's vital need for "essential" fatty acids, healthy fats and oils also impart a longer lasting sense of satiety, quite the opposite of refined carbs, so don't fall into the trap of eliminating whole food groups with the intent of losing weight. ALL basic food groups (protein, carbs, and fats) have to be consumed in <u>balanced moderation</u> for optimum health and attaining proper weight.

MYTH: "CALORIES IN vs. CALORIES OUT": It goes something like this: calculate your basal metabolic rate (an estimation at best of the – identical - calories you burn every day just "keeping the lights on" - staying alive), add the additional calories you burn exercising (based on wildly inaccurate exercise tables and cardio machines, not to mention not always factoring in intensity) and balance with calories consumed (based on exact counts of … guestimates and downright wrong data), and you end up … *with a mess!* Come on, if it were that easy obesity wouldn't exist, dietary technicians, food & exercise gurus, and a host of diet-advice companies would be out of business. It's not enough that any single of the above mentioned factors that go into calculating your caloric needs vs. expenditures has a sizeable margin of error. Once you add them all up the resulting numbers could be all over the place – including right on target if you are lottery-type lucky. And there is a lot more trouble out there, since they have messed with our hormone systems, rendering our usually reliable 'compass' to stay on a healthy weight course nearly useless.

Still, the biggest problem with the "calorie in – calorie out" fairy tale is the mistaken belief that just power-walking those extra 30 minutes a day (or burning calories in other ways) will absolve you of your need to know when to say "when", make healthy food choices, use proper portion sizes, consume the same or fewer calories spread out over more meals, and eat healthy, balanced foods. As you get more active, your body will eventually ask for more calories, and if you give in and furnish it the additional calories you burned during exercising you are no further ahead as far as reducing your weight is concerned (although you'll still reap certain health benefits from the extra activity). Once you have reached your desired goal, obviously you want to consume only as many calories as you expand every day, which will vary from one day to the next.

MYTH: "I CAN'T COOK HEALTHY MEALS – I DON'T KNOW HOW TO COOK": So what's wrong with that? *Not knowing how to cook is probably a good thing!* Traditional cooking relies too much on "over"- cooking anyway: battering, deep-frying, covering up foods with fatty sauces, adding layers of fat or sodium or sugar, and in general turning healthy raw ingredients into nutritionally inferior meals. Whenever the total is <u>less</u> than the sum of its parts we have done the exact opposite of what preparing a meal should be all about which is combining foods to arrive at a balanced meal where the total is <u>more</u> than the sum of its parts.

Here's a typical meal that illustrates that point. Nobody would think twice about ordering a "healthy" dinner of pasta primavera at a local Italian restaurant, right? And of course you'll order the (healthy) salad first, and they always serve hot garlic bread with butter the moment you sit down. When you add it all up you had a great evening at an Italian trattoria – and an unbalanced, inferior meal: processed white grains served with …. more processed white grains, some token vegetables (and the iceberg lettuce doesn't count), and lots of fat, some good (olive oil), some not so good (butter). Not exactly balanced or healthy (where's the protein, for one?). Instead you could have ordered a vegetable - (brown) rice pilaf with a small side of (wild-caught) salmon or trout or seared tuna, and nibbled peanuts from the bar instead of that serving of white bread covered with butter: now you have a quality protein (fish), legumes (peanuts) and whole grains (brown rice – a quality, low-glycemic carbohydrate; no extra charge for fiber) complementing each other to form another complete protein, and vegetables (in the risotto; more fiber); salad optional (go for spinach or mixed greens).

And you can do even better at home. Surely you can sauté (or bake in aluminum foil) a piece of fish in peanut oil (or pop open a can of kippered herring), steam a vegetable of your choice (or a freezer-pack vegetable medley), or pour some healthy ready-made dressing (low sodium, low fat, and no sugar) over a pre-packaged salad mix (iceberg lettuce doesn't count). Cooking rice is no mystery either: just add 2-3 cups of water to 1 cup of brown rice and let simmer without a top until all the water is gone. Either the rice is done (mission accomplished!) or you'll add some more water and try again when that has evaporated. Or, take a short-cut and toast a few slices of gluten-free or whole-grain bread ("Food for Life"™; "Ezekiel"™; "Alvarado Street Bakery"™) and serve with extra virgin olive oil instead of butter. There – you had control of all the ingredients, know 100% what's on your plate (never a sure thing in a restaurant), and had a meal nutritionally superior to "what's for dinner" at over 90% of restaurants. And you can pronounce and spell all the ingredients of your meal, and save some money too

Take a similar approach to baked potatoes (plain; cook in oven for 30-45 minutes depending on size; 390-400° should do it), delicious root vegetables (taro, parsnips, boniata, malanga, beet, etc.), alternative grains (quinoa, millet, teff, endless varieties of brown rice), pasture-raised eggs (maybe you can't cook that perfect omelet, but anybody can hard-boil an egg which is better for you anyway – no added fat, and just one egg; skip the egg-cheaters), and other vegetables (steamed is best; use the steaming water - containing a lot of nutrients – for your next batch of rice or soups). And you can always super-charge a meal with a combination of legumes and nuts and/or seeds, which are easily added to salads or just eaten plain. They can make a healthy, small snack all by themselves: lentils, chickpeas, beans, crunchy roasted green peas (or wasabi peas – take a trip to the nearest Oriental supermarket), peanuts combined with various nuts and seeds. The combinations are endless. Add crunchy roasted vegetable chips (watch for fat content), fresh fruit, experiment with fresh herbs (cooked, or just sprinkled fresh on top – it doesn't get any easier than that), add flaxseed meal (1-3 tablespoons) to your daily routine, and you have a solid foundation for a healthy diet. Sure, there's other things you need (a changing variety of protein sources, a bigger variety of vegetables and fruit, some tofu and tempeh, other essential fatty acids, some supplements, etc.), but already you have a solid foundation upon which you can build – as long as you keep a vigilant eye on portion sizes.

DIET MYTH: fruit is healthy and low in calories, yet high in bulk. Eating lots of it will get the weight off. This is also known as the "more is better" myth.

FACT: nice try. Yes, fruits are healthy foods and should be an important part of your diet. But if you eat too much of them you <u>still</u> get too much sugar – which can make you gain weight. Any excess fructose (especially the kind that is added to processed foods) can raise blood lipid levels. Oooops! Fruit should be <u>part</u> of a balanced diet, and too much of a good thing risks sugar overload and excess calories. Remember, fruit should be consumed in lesser quantities than vegetables, so veggies first, fruit second.

DIET MYTH: switching to artificial, non-caloric sweeteners will save a lot of calories, and the weight will melt away.

FACT: if it were that easy …. obesity would be virtually unknown, or at least there'd be a lot less of it. Sadly, we cannot fool our bodies that easily. While you save 30 or more calories for every cup of tea or coffee that you'll sweeten with artificial sweeteners instead of sugar, your body is "on to you" and feels cheated out of the sugar fix the artificial sweeteners promised. So it asks for more. And if you feed it real sugar instead, the crash after the spike will result in more sugar cravings, so you can't win either way, and get addicted either way. As a matter of fact there is evidence that people who consume a lot of artificial sweeteners (usually in the form of diet soft drinks) tend to be more overweight than people who do not use them at all. Certainly there are many other factors involved: probably people who avoid artificial sweeteners make better lifestyle choices in general (exercising, keeping a constant weight, better diet, etc.), but it is probably safe to assume that non-caloric sweeteners, while helpful for certain uses in limited quantities, generally speaking are not the "get out of [the fat-] jail free card". Read up on sweeteners in the chapter "The Sweet Tooth".

DIET MYTH: people who work out a lot (think marathon runners, Ironmen, ultra cyclists, etc.) can eat whatever they want, and as much as they want. This myth just won't go away. Sure, if you are a world-class decathlete (in the prime of your life) competing at the world championship in Berlin you may get away with eating apple strudel every day – and then go out and set a world record. But A. that's an exception, and B. chances are that doesn't describe YOU. And of course that athlete didn't get good enough to compete at the highest levels on a diet of apple strudel. YOU could easily become one of those ultra-fit cyclists who average over 100 miles a week – and are 50 lbs. overweight! They are out there, and most likely their downfall is beer or greasy food.

FACT: it just doesn't work that way. Too much saturated fat will still clog up otherwise healthy arteries, too many simple carbohydrates will still only supply empty calories, and too many calories of any kind can still pack on the pounds. Refined sugar products are performance drainers of the worst kind. If you think you really deserve that big slice of death-by-chocolate cake (900 – or so unhealthy calories) you'd have run nearly 10 miles that day to make up for that sugar bomb. And that only burns the calories and doesn't address the sub-standard food now in your system. Treating yourself to that latte every morning (on top of your regular breakfast), and a super-sized lunch every day will take a lot of sweat equity to burn off, apart from the fact that the empty calories will be ill-suited to give your body the premium fuel it needs. Bottom Line: you still have to make good choices at the dinner table (and breakfast, and lunch) and pay attention to portion sizes.

RECOVERY MYTH 1: After a strenuous / long workout or race you should consume a carbohydrate snack (or a 4:1 carbohydrate-protein snack) 30-60 minutes after exercising.

FACT 1: *if you wait that long before you feed your screaming-for-food body, the recovery train has long ago left the station,* and your body will hustle all day (and longer) to catch up. You need recovery fuel *within minutes,* not up to an hour later. Don't feel like eating right after exercising? Find something you can stomach very shortly after your workout, or try a recovery drink – anything that you can consume sooner, rather than later. You can train your body to do that. It will make a world of difference how you feel immediately after the workout, the rest of the day, and when you do your next workout.

FACT 2: carbs or that magic 4:1 carb/ protein formula will work just fine for a moderate-effort, moderate-duration workout. And a brisk walk around the block doesn't need anything special right afterwards, so skip that sugary alligator drink. But if you are exhausted from a marathon, triathlon, long swim session, a serious iron-pumping session, or any major physical effort you need a serious serving of quality protein – right then and there. You want to jump-start that muscle repair job with the right tools – protein, with some carbs added. And that is one of the rare times where a protein shake designed for rapid recovery may just be the best food to put into your system. No, it isn't health food, and most high protein recovery products have their share of less-than-pure ingredients, but in this case those concerns should take a backseat. Designed for a purpose – recovery – these shakes *work*. Then, an hour or so later you should follow it up with *real* food, in the form of a balanced meal.

RECOVERY MYTH 2: chocolate milk is a great post-workout recovery food.

FACT: putting 25% of your daily "requirement" of saturated fat, plus 30 grams (!) of sugar, and 25 mg of cholesterol in one very unhealthy package does not add up to a healthy-*anytime* snack, and certainly not at a time when <u>premium recovery fuel</u> is called for. Sounds like a dairy infomercial to me.

You can do better than that – much better. Muscle Milk™ Light has <u>half</u> the saturated fat, only <u>2 g</u> of sugar, and only <u>5 mg</u> of cholesterol. How about all-important protein content for muscle repair? Milk: 8 g – M.M.L.: 25 g. Bottom Line: this isn't even close. Other excellent choices would be "Muscle Milk Light No Sugar Added"™ after a shorter, but still intense exercise session (only 100 calories but still <u>double</u> the protein of chocolate milk), Recoverite™ from Hammer Nutrition, EAS Myoplex™, or one of the "AMP" products from GNC, like "Amplified Wheybolic Extreme 60". Yes, they do contain dairy products (usually whey and casein) – but you save a lot of unnecessary calories and saturated fats, and these products are widely available; another "lesser of two evils" situation. Better choices would be plant based protein supplements, like pea protein, brown rice protein, etc. or egg protein. There's even a mixed vegan protein powder out there, made by a company called Genuine Health™. Soy protein powder, if derived from organic (hence non-GMO) soybeans is another, more readily available option, as long as you don't rely on it exclusively and/or in large quantities. There are other excellent muscle repair and recovery products out there, but watch total calories and sugar content. And don't forget to include <u>real</u> food with those ready-made recovery shakes (a banana or other fruit, raisins, dates, a small PB&J sandwich – if done right; etc.) and then have a balanced meal an hour or two later.

RESISTANCE TRAINING (WEIGHT ROOM) MYTH: "I don't want to pump iron since I don't want to bulk up".

FACT: HA! You could only wish you were this lucky. Unless you are in your prime (in your 20-ies, maybe 30-ies), and plan to shed blood, sweat and tears for several hours 5-6 days of the week in the gym, chances are slim to none this will happen to you. Even then a healthy dose of good genes – and the right chromosomes – are often required to bulk up beyond what most people would consider "normal". So by all means, hit that gym twice or 3 times per week for a whole body workout for all the benefits and no drawbacks. Low weight / high reps, when combined with 'meaningful' cardio workouts will get you strong without bulking up.

Read up on this **"fountain of youth"** in the "Staying Healthy Longer" chapter.

"ANTI-OXIDANTS IN SHINING ARMOR RIDING TO THE RESCUE TO DEFEND AGAINST EVIL FREE RADICALS" MYTH:

FACT? I am not so sure about that. Think back 50 or 100 or more years. Even then, trim, fit athletes were considered a picture of good health who enjoyed life longer, had a better quality of life, and had fewer medical issues. Judging by all the anti-oxidant hype jumping off fortified foods packages these days one would have to think that the then unknown (and therefore unchecked) free radicals created by exercise stress would have ravaged these seemingly healthy people. That didn't happen; weekend warriors and competitive athletes alike did not keel over in large numbers to be buried in mass graves.

So how did they manage to survive this post-exercise onslaught of free radicals? Maybe by training their bodies to deal with them – assisted by a healthy diet of vegetables, fruit, legumes, nuts, root vegetables, quality proteins, etc, all of which were abundant in natural anti-oxidants. And since their caloric requirements were higher than their sedentary contemporaries, they ate more of everything, and most of that was healthy & wholesome. Back in those days more vegetables and fruit were locally grown, were more likely to be organic (or at least less polluted), and the little meat that was eaten back then roamed a pasture near you only a few days, or hours, before ending up on their dinner plates. Contrast that to produce grown in depleted soils these days, on huge mono-culture farms, and meats from animals that were fed an unnatural cocktail of industrial feed (sometimes with ground-up animal parts mixed in, counter to the fact that these animals are strict plant eaters- maybe it's not the cows that have gone mad!) and it's easy to see that we are not giving our bodies the best tools to deal with "evil free radicals". At best these foods have a fraction of the necessary components or quantities of a healthy diet, but lack the 'whole package' of known and unknown compounds beneficial to human health (which help repair temporary exercise-induced damage). So if, collectively, we spent more of our food dollar on organic produce, pasture-raised protein sources, wild-caught fish, and bought at local farmers' markets, maybe we could save spending all that money on super anti-oxidant berry juice from the Amazon jungle, or "fortified" faux health food. The only vegetables or fruit that don't have natural anti-oxidants are the ones that have not found a generous P.R. agent yet or couldn't afford to be "scientifically" tested! Not much lobbying or advertising money out there for testing and hyping the benefits of beets, parsnips or taro roots.

Chances are good that a moderate amount of "anti-oxidant" supplements will not do any harm, so if it makes you feel better, go ahead. But your best bet still lies with "real" foods – and avoiding **inflammatory foods**, such as saturated fats, sugars, salt, alcohol and most highly processed food products. Also, recent research seems to confirm that raging free radicals may have a positive effect on your body, by conditioning your body to fight them and neutralizing them. Maybe we should think of exercise-strengthened bodies like we think of strong immune systems, strengthened over years of fighting infectious diseases vs. living in a sterile bubble. No doubt further research will clarify – or confuse – the subject further. Stay tuned, keep exercising, and don't sit around.

HELPFUL HINTS ... AND PITFALLS (to avoid)

What is the single most important thing in your life?

- Your children?
- Your spouse?
- Your parents?
- Friends?
- Religion?
- Your career?
- Money / Financial Security?
- Reaching your potential?

These are all worthy and important things – but not as important as your **health.** Without it, everything else can become meaningless or impossible to achieve.

- You are of no help to your children if you are sick, or in the hospital, or immobile, or need more help than you can provide. And you want to be around when they get married, have children and grandchildren, no?

- How can you extend your love to your spouse, and brighten his/her day, if you are in pain and/or discomfort, probably resulting in a burden on him or her? At the very least you'll be cranky and no fun to be around. And in the worst case scenario, what will become of your spouse in the event of your early demise?

- How can you help your (ageing) parents, if you need help yourself?

- Religion can be the salvation for some people – but Alzheimer's disease will make this a moot point.

- Your career will be cut short of your most productive years if you are unable to perform at your peak abilities when you get there. And like it or not, overweight, but competent people are sometimes over-looked when it's time for promotions. Life isn't fair.

- Money … can't buy happiness they say – and it sure can't buy quality or quantity of life. And a serious disease can drain most people's savings frighteningly fast.

- In order to reach your potential (intellectually, athletically, financially) you have to be on top of your game. "Sound mind in a sound body", and such, remember?

Your health takes priority over everything else in life.

Assuming you bought this book to address your weight problem, what is your biggest challenge?

What is the single biggest obstacle that keeps most people from getting their weight into the "desirable" range: <u>addiction to food</u> – but you knew that. What you may not realize however is that the addiction to <u>sugary</u> foods may have the most negative effect on your health, and it's also the hardest to overcome. So while there are addictions to other foods (favorite snacks, greasy burgers, salty foods, high-fat foods, and more) chances are the most important thing many people must do is …

Kick the sugar habit

Making the addiction to sugar (empty 'white' calories) even more insidious is the fact that just like any addiction, giving in (having that one sweet treat) only leads to a renewed desire to have another "hit". And calorie-free sweeteners (low-cal, really) may be even worse in that regard! There is no way around it – sugar is the drug that you have to eliminate from your system. And yes, it is possible. Since most likely just reading this will send some people into sugar-withdrawal depressions – thinking of nothing else but sweet treats – let's try this exercise: make a list of all the (healthy) salty foods and snacks, including those without any added sugar (fruits, veggies, etc.). Go ahead; write them all down, all your non-sugary favorites. NOW would be a good time, so put this book down and make that list.

O.K. – finished? You should have come up with a pretty good list of many mouth-watering foods that are healthy (scratch off all fast-food fare, pretzels, Doritos, chips, etc. – be honest with yourself). From now on only think about all the foods on this list, and no other! You like peanuts – now you can enjoy them (in moderation) since you will eliminate all the sugar-filled empty calories. And peanuts will give you that feeling of satiety longer and avoid cravings for more, and more, and then some. Same goes for other legumes – think wasabi peas, chickpeas, lentils, beans, etc. Same goes for nuts, which you have always avoided because "they have too many calories". No they don't – if you have moderate amounts as a meal, not several handfuls *in addition to* an unhealthy meal. Ditto for avocadoes, carrot salad, veggie snacks, etc. The moment you think of any sweet thing you would love to have as your next snack, take a look at this list and have one of your "salty favorites" instead. Nothing on that list sounds tempting? Good – that means that you are not hungry at all, but have a sugar-hit craving, and the best way to deal with it – if you can't ignore it – is having a small salty snack, or vegetable or fruit.

Trust me on this – **kicking the sugar habit will show positive results**! It **will** start a downward spiral of weight loss, especially when combined with increased physical activity, and when making good dietary choices as outlined in this book. And this step you can take NOW, for immediate results, so before you have another sweet-anything, re-read the "Sweet Tooth" chapter.

Your second biggest enemy

This one is not your fault. It's the 25- minute or so delay from your stomach to tell your brain that you are full and really don't want to eat any more. I call it a human design flaw, one we have to live with – and one we can outsmart. How? If you use good portion control for all your meals and snacks (see "The Basics" for details) you will have properly sized meals, and chances are good you will not feel "full" when you are done. That's good! What is not good is going for seconds, or dessert! Instead, consider the possibility that you are really full already (alien as it may seem at the time) and your brain just has not gotten that message yet.

NOW is the time for a new approach:

Start using your timing device: promise yourself that you will have that dessert or second serving that you crave – after 25 minutes, when time's up. Anything will do: a Timex™ watch, egg timer, alarm clock, cell phone, or any other timing device.

O.K. – time's up, are you really still hungry? We are not talking about cravings – which should have vanished also, but about hunger. Be honest with yourself! When in doubt take the "apple test": if you don't care to have an apple (or asparagus, or any other food you like, but don't crave), but would love to have that piece of chocolate (or second servings of anything) it's not hunger. Chances are that you really felt sated after 25 minutes or so, and that any additional food lost all its attraction. Don't force it – you are now in a great position to just walk away from food, and stop thinking about it – except maybe thinking about your next meal in 3-4 hours. Better yet, chances are you will have forgotten about eating altogether! **Practice it, use it, do it.**

Nobody will make fun of you – and if they do, they'll stop laughing (and be impressed) when a few weeks or months later the weight is coming down, down, down, and everybody wonders where you found the willpower to make it happen.

"I have over-eaten terribly at that last meal – help!"

Over-eating occasionally can be a good thing!

1. It happens to the best of us – and re-enforces a lesson to not do it again, since we typically remember for a long time how bad we felt afterwards. We all need reminders like this sometime.
2. How many problems can you think of that will go away by doing ... *nothing*? That's right, now that you stopped eating and surveyed the damage, help is already on the way – in the form of doing no more harm (you stopped eating), and waiting. Sure you can take a walk, or spin easy, or do any other form of light exercise to help speed the process along, but even just doing nothing will eventually right things.

Having said that, of course it is important to:

1. Stop eating (the sooner the better – don't heap misery upon misery). Don't fall into the trap of "I lost it – might as well go for that 2nd – and 3rd – piece of pie".
2. Make sure that this over-eating 'incidence' is a very rare exception

And if you feel really, really guilty this could be a good time to clear out your fridge and pantry of food items of dubious nutritional value that got you in trouble in the first place.

The devil is in the details

PERSON A: A "Peanut Butter & Jelly sandwiches is junk food"
PERSON B: "A Peanut Butter & Jelly sandwich is health food".

So who is right?
BOTH!

170

Here's how "A" & "B" look at the old PB&J sandwich, from their perspective.

PERSON A makes a PB&J sandwich with pearly-white accordion bread (empty calories, stripped of any meaningful nutritional value, with many – 20 or more – non-nutritive mystery substances added, expiration date in the distant future), Skip-It peanut butter (with added sugar, hydrogenated fats, and possibly preservatives, conditioners and fillers), and commercial jelly (mostly sugar, or corn syrup or HFCS – high fructose corn syrup – or, if you are "lucky", all three) – more empty calories, with the added hazard of attacking your teeth even harder and faster than refined flour products alone. This is truly junk food, masquerading as a "wholesome" all-American traditional food. To make matters worse, consumption of this high glycemic sandwich will result in the familiar sugar rush followed by a crash thereafter, and cravings for more simple carbohydrates – as well as cravings for real nutrients that the "A" sandwich didn't provide. I just hope "person A" doesn't put this kind of "food" into his or her children's lunch boxes. Ritalin anyone?

PERSON B makes a PB&J sandwich with real bread (let's say, Food for Life™ gluten-free bread, or other real whole grain bread), Laura Scudder's™ all natural peanut butter, and either sugar-free or fruit-juice sweetened preserves. Let's see - whole, gluten-free grains combined with natural legumes (peanuts) form a quality complete protein, peanut butter also contributes healthy essential fatty acids, and NSA (no-sugar-added) preserves add good carbohydrates. And the "B" sandwich has a much lower glycemic index, and – no surprise there – **tastes a whole lot better** too. That's a pretty good resume to qualify for "healthy food" status, I would say. So which person are you?

Bottom Line: check the facts and all the (nutritional) details carefully before jumping to conclusions. Many "healthy-looking" products (even entire companies) count on their customers' ignorance to never look beyond the faux health façade.

Beware traditional dietary "cookie cutter" advice
(No matter where it comes from)

FOR EXAMPLE .....

FACT: turmeric is truly a miracle food – just ask the people on the Indian sub-continent who have adopted it as their own and liberally add it to many dishes of their justly famous cuisines. For one, prostrate cancer is virtually unknown among Indian men, and it has well-known anti-inflammatory properties - take note, arthritis sufferers. Turmeric, and its active ingredient curcumin, are also believed to help digestive disorders, have detoxifying, antiseptic and antibacterial properties, and may even show promise in treating Alzheimer's disease. We probably haven't heard the end of turmeric's health potential yet, so stay tuned.

STANDARD COOKIE-CUTTER ADVICE: "Sprinkle some turmeric into water when boiling rice".

PROBLEM: Sprinkle? Sure, if you eat *several* pounds of rice with *every* meal you might just get enough turmeric to result in faint health benefits. No, all those few sprinkles spread out over one or more servings of rice will get you is a hint of color – and probably no measurable health benefits.

WHAT YOU NEED: **liberal** amounts of turmeric! Indians aren't shy about using it beyond a "sprinkle", and you can smell their turmeric and curry–flavored dishes from a mile away. Even then, turmeric is poorly absorbed (*double that rice* with the "sprinkles" in it that you would have to eat ...) and needs black pepper to perform its various healthy jobs in the human body. Luckily Indian dishes are not known for insufficient black pepper either, so keep that pepper grinder handy. How much is "liberal"? Let your senses of smell and taste be your guide – keep adding turmeric until it is overpowering, then dial it back until you have a still-rich, yellow-tainted, delicious meal. And of course turmeric doesn't grow in cans or bags or jars, so find some turmeric root in your local Oriental supermarket, peel it and add to vegetables, stews, meats, eggs, etc. Still, turmeric powder provides a lot of the same health benefits, so avail yourself of that more convenient option if the root is not available or convenient.

What's not to like about a (cheap) food ingredient that will improve your health and introduces you to a new taste experience at the same time? Can't stand the thought of eating Indian-style food? Well, you are missing out, but you could at least try some turmeric (curcumin) supplements, with additional black pepper (or piperine). Unfortunately isolating active ingredients to obtain health benefits attributed to the whole, natural food has an undistinguished record of success. And while reasonable quantities of fresh or powdered turmeric are considered safe for consumption, you may want to check with your health care provider before starting a new supplement regime.

.

STANDARD COOKIE-CUTTER ADVICE: "You can eat healthy meals at fast food restaurants, and some junk food can actually be good for you". **Don't fall for it.**

Here is how it started: since the Double M.I. Burger has a gazillion calories, enough saturated fats and cholesterol to cover your "needs" for a whole week, and sodium levels to justify its name, certainly the Slim-Jim Grilled Chicken Sandwich at a mere (?) 550 calories, and only a day's worth of fat, is super healthy in comparison. Right – as long as we conveniently ignore the fact that the chicken lived a short, miserable life on a c.c. farm, and in death will impart to *you* all the chemicals, drugs, growth hormones and antibiotics it was forced to consume. People also tend to ignore that this sub-par piece of protein (probably grilled with a coating of cheap vegetable oil) is served on a bun made from the finest bleached, over-processed white flour money can buy, which has been robbed of most of its nutritional value, and – if you are "lucky" – is served with iceberg lettuce, which still qualifies as a healthy vegetable to some people, but isn't. This concept of "comparatively good" makes a plain old Smacker's Bar healthy, since, hey – it's not deep fried (like they sell at the rodeo – no, really!).

Sugar Bomb Brand Cereal anyone? Heck, now that it has psyllium added to the over-processed mix it qualifies as a heart-healthy food! It's a steep, slippery slope, and you'd be best off avoiding it altogether. How about treating yourself to an occasional small piece of cheesecake to avoid being overcome by craving attacks during which you demolish the whole cake? Sure, one piece vs. the whole cake would appear to be an improvement – IF you can stop at that one piece. Since sugar and all simple carbohydrate cravings act like drugs on your body you may find it difficult to stop after that one piece. Consider this: has anybody ever suggested you treat yourself to one cigarette every once in a while, or one joint – all so you don't start chain smoking a whole pack? Enough said.

THE TRUTH OF THE MATTER: **"Good-for-you junk food" is an oxymoron.** Yes, there are *less unhealthy* choices that can be made in just about any restaurant, and there are *less unhealthy* junk foods than others, but no matter how you look at these *less unhealthy* "foods", they become no healthier by contrast to even unhealthier options. No more so than an overweight person is likely to look (or feel) slim or healthy when standing next to an obese person.

COURSE OF ACTION: don't settle for *slightly less unhealthy.* You will reap slightly noticeable results, improve your health marginally, if at all, get frustrated by the lack of progress, and abort your attempts to meaningful changes.

Dining Out

THIS IS DANGEROUS TERRITORY. Making healthy, quality food choices of dishes that have been minimally processed in restaurants is a stiff challenge. Your first and best defense is not going out at all. Not very practical – after all, dining out is one of the great pleasures in life one should not deny oneself, and sometimes it is a necessity. Maybe reducing the number of meals you eat out is a more realistic goal. Whenever possible, choose the type of restaurant wisely. "You get what you pay for" holds especially true for dining out (with the honorable exception of some great ethnic eateries which usually offer great value for money), and by that I don't mean that the top-of-the-line restaurants will serve the healthiest food – but the cheapest restaurant, in general, will serve the least healthy fare. ("Who said fast-food restaurants?"). They did not get big by offering top-notch quality (usually expensive) food items for ridiculously little money. We all know instinctively that there is something inherently wrong with a burger selling for $1.00, when a single apple at the supermarket can cost more than that. Sure, one can make (relatively) healthy choices at any eatery, but skinless c.c. chicken breast and iceberg lettuce with a canned dressing containing too many unpronounceable ingredients will sustain you for a few hours, but add very little to the health bottom line.

When deciding on a restaurant, ask yourself not only how unhealthy the fare there might be (starting with the "Triple Threat" of too much sodium, cheap fat, refined sugars, or carbohydrates), but also think of what all you are **not** getting:

- Green, leafy vegetables?
- Cruciferous vegetables?
- Root vegetables?
- Fresh fruit?
- Quality protein from pasture-raised animals or non-GMO plant sources?
- Legumes?
- Herbs and spices?
- Fiber?
- Nuts or seeds?
- Omega-3 and other essential fatty acids (corn oil, soy oil, cottonseed oil don't count!)?
- Brown rice, or other whole grains?

That doesn't leave a lot of restaurants, right? Certainly not the chain outlets that offer high-gloss menus with dishes that look picture-book perfect – and fresh off an assembly line, which they basically are. So again, make the least unhealthy choices. Your best bet usually lies not with chain restaurants (unless you are lucky and find one of the few-and-far-between exceptions; Chipotle Grill™ comes to mind) but those where the owner stakes his or her reputation and livelihood on them, an owner who buys local fresh ingredients and recognizes that over-processing fresh ingredients only dilutes the taste. In these places you will find many of the above-mentioned healthy foods that are "endangered species" in most mainstream dining establishments. Try to find <u>authentic</u> Oriental restaurants; there, most foods are minimally processed (sautéed vs. deep-fried, steamed vs. boiled, healthy seasonings vs. heavy sauces for inferior protein to hide under, etc.), light and appropriately portioned (vs. super-sized). Experiment, make healthy choices, have fun – and eat at a variety of restaurants if you must dine out – or just plain feel like it. And always keep in mind that we have yet to hear from a centenarian who credits dining out a lot for his or her longevity. Ponder that thought.

A special mention should be made of the perils of patronizing **buffets**. It is nearly impossible for anybody to make smart food choices and limit portion sizes at all-you-can-eat buffets. The tendency to try just one more thing proves that too much variety (at one time) can work against you, as you overload your plate and/or return for 2nd, 3rd, or even 4th servings. Sure, an all-you-can-eat salad bar sounds like a healthy way to dine out, but reality is often quite different: calorie-laden salad dressings, little quality protein, unbalanced meals, and excess caloric intake are serious risks that can derail most people's best intentions. If you are stuck at a buffet for whatever reason, I would suggest to take only ONE trip to the buffet, assemble a small, balanced meal on your plate, ask yourself if this looks like a normal sized meal (600 calories max!), and then add no more, and never, ever go back for seconds. "Getting your money's worth" at the expense of your health is short-sighted thinking. And keep in mind that these establishments are in it to make a profit, so above average consumption has to be offset by – you guessed it – cheap ingredients.

Equally dangerous as buffets are **parties** (think Christmas time). Don't let the intended purpose of having fun, celebrating, meeting good friends and making new ones deteriorate into eating orgies that you'll regret long after those good party memories have faded. Some people who dread these gatherings make matters worse by starving themselves beforehand "to make room" for the excessive amounts of foods that no doubt will be too good to resist. A better strategy would be to have a small (healthy) snack an hour or so before you arrive at those food-laden tables, and at the very least you will not be starving and vulnerable to "first available" foods of questionable nutritional value (chips & dips, crackers & cheese, etc.) Chances are you've lost your appetite, can mix and mingle first without being sidetracked by your growling stomach and will not make a mad dash for the food line. Make that "pre-party" snack a filling, yet low-calorie choice, like a cup of miso soup, asparagus, carrot salad, a slice of avocado, an apple or some other piece of fruit, a large (healthy) beverage, etc., and you will get the additional help of the full-feeling that these foods provide. Later on during the party, by all means enjoy some of the foods available in moderation (making smart choices), but since you were not starving to begin with, chances are excellent that you feel great during and afterwards without the caloric "hangover".

Dining In

THIS CAN BE DANGEROUS TERRITORY TOO!

For one, portion control is up to you now, which can be a blessing (as in the case of super-sized meals in restaurants) or a hazard (you can overload your plate just as easily yourself – and 'seconds' are only a few steps away at the stove top or refrigerator). It's what YOU make of it! Use your instincts when putting together a meal: put it all on one plate (or some items on a small side plate, like salad) and gauge the 'offerings' to double-check if the portion size looks about right for that particular meal (200 min / 600 max calories).

Again – **be honest with yourself!** You may guess wrong at first. If your "eyes were bigger than your stomach", just put down that eating utensil and **stop**! You can always have the leftovers at a later time – or never, but don't over-eat just to be a good girl (or boy) and finish what's served. If your meal was too small, well, that's a good problem, because you'll stop eating anyway (I hope – for your sake!) and have that next meal sooner. Eventually you'll get a feel for proper portion sizing that is just right for you at any given point, something no calorie-counting dietician can do for you in the long run.

Another trap to avoid: putting anything but portion-sized foods on your plate or the table. That means no huge bags of chips ("can't just eat one", remember?), no buckets of butter (which shouldn't be in your house in the first place; use small amounts of "Earth Balance"™ instead), no jars of mayonnaise, preserves or peanut butter (if it has more than 2 ingredients and oil does not separate don't buy it), no big casserole begging for 2nd servings, no family-style dining where the good conversations and the servings of food never stop. None-such – remember you are on a mission to lose what can be life-threatening extra pounds, and these "restrictions" (which become second nature quickly) are the kind you can live with. When you get up from a meal and feel energized rather than full and sluggish you have succeeded and won one small battle in the war. It should feel so good that you want to win many more battles, and never go back to old habits.

Maybe you need some crutches

Assuming you'll give up a lot of familiar foods that really aren't advancing your health, you'll feel deprived sooner or later and need some help to adjust to that change. Think of 'reformed' smokers who run around with a toothpick in their mouths all day long, or start chewing gum. Crutches are not a good thing, and I do not recommend them, but if used wisely and for limited periods of time, there is a place for them. Just beware the danger of getting addicted to them and undoing all or some of the good they may have done in the first place.

Speaking of (sugar-free) chewing gum - it can be an effective tool to kick your sugar habit, and stop snacking after meals too. And of course there are all those health claims that want to convince you it is an important part of your daily oral hygiene. True to a point, as long as you restrict yourself to an occasional (one) piece after a meal. But, it can become counterproductive if you chew a pack a day! For one, there are enough artificial ingredients in sugar-free gum to keep big chemical plants in business. For another, most of them contain aspartame (just say no!). And thirdly, almost all of them contain other artificial sweeteners that can cause stomach problems. Gas and diarrhea will not improve the quality of your life, or of anybody near you. The same holds true for sugar-free mints, candy and all other snacks, so limit yourself to the occasional consumption of these mutated foods, or better yet avoid them altogether.

Diet soft drinks are another crutch: great if you wean yourself off "fully leaded" soft drinks (basically carbonated sugar water), but they will almost certainly not help you lose weight in the long run. Remember, you can't trick your smart body into thinking it just got a serving of sweet carbs, and it will keep asking for the "real thing" – quality carbs. Plus, you'll tend to retain water whenever you consume fizzy drinks, and I don't even want to go into the more serious health issues of soft drinks at this point. Can't shake the habit? I thought so too, until I forced myself to give up this unhealthy vice. The amazing outcome: after switching to green teas, fruit and herb teas, and drinking more water of course, I lost all interest in carbonated soft drinks, most all of which started to taste very artificial – which they are of course.

About "fruit and vegetables"

Yes, they are healthy, and yes, they should take up the most space on your plate, but I move to make a subtle change in that term. Let's just call it in order of priorities, and refer to plant foods as **"vegetables and fruit"**. After all vegetables and root vegetables are the natural foods that do all the things fruit can do – but do not carry the risk of adding to a sugar overload. That doesn't mean we should eliminate fruit from our diet (or quality proteins, essential fatty acids, etc.), but vegetables simply deserve top billing.

ORGANIC foods – are they really worth the "price of admission"?

Entire books have been written on that subject, and this will not be one of them. I'll give you the short version instead.

- Yes, organic foods are invariably better for you than their conventional counterparts. You'll find references throughout this book about their nutritional qualities and benefits. And "better for you" does not always mean "better tasting", although most of the time they will. A fresh, local, crisp 'conventional' apple in season can taste better than an organic, imported apple – but chances are the former will still be nutritionally inferior to the latter.

- No, chances are you won't buy "all organic" from now on. I don't. For one, some foods just aren't available everywhere in organic versions, for another some of them are prohibitively expensive, and lastly, some conventional foods can be nearly as nutritious as the organic version. See comments on the "Food Rankings Chart" for more details.

- The good news: a lot of organic produce has become very affordable – on par with conventionally grown versions – so some of the highly polluted or nutrient-poor foods can be avoided altogether.

- More good news: buying organic assures you that only non-genetically modified crops are used. Since the verdict is still out on the safety of these altered plants you won't be the guinea pig to find out one way or another.

- Oh, and they can't use sewage on organic soils either, which is a comforting thought next time you eat raw vegetables or fruit (but you still have to wash them first).

- No worries about dangerous chemicals in your food supply either. Or antibiotics or hormone residues. And vegetarian cows raised organically aren't fed a non-vegetarian, sometimes cannibalistic, diet either. Try not to think about that too long – just reach for the organic version.

- A lot of locally-grown produce and meat or eggs from locally-raised livestock are organic in all but name, since many small farmers, "hobby farmers", small co-ops, etc. simply do not want to add the cost of getting certified to their products. Chances are there's a farmer's market in your area – check it out and discover new foods and a better alternative than the nearest hyper mart.

- Foods that are not necessarily organic that you should not compromise on: wild-caught vs. farm-raised (with possible exception to "responsibly farmed" option – do your homework), pasture-raised vs. "anything else" (terms like "cage-free", and "free-range", etc. have been devalued by clever food corporations who found the loopholes), and over-processed, "de-natured" food-like products. And produce with the highest pesticide loads (refer to the comments on the Food Rankings chart) should be avoided if at all possible.

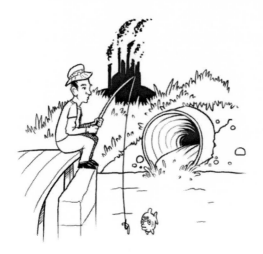

So you don't think it matters where your protein comes from ....

Would you eat this 'catch of the day'? Farm-raised could be worse.

- So organic eggs from pasture-raised chicken cost upward of $4.00 p. dozen? And organic strawberries go for $1.00-$3.00 more p. pound than 'conventional'? That's still only pennies per egg, and a dozen eggs can last a person for 2 weeks, and the strawberries make for several servings – all for skipping one multissimo-grandissimo beverage at your local Mega-Bucks? Seems like a bargain to me. Along those lines ....

- *Do a little soul searching:* in the U.S., people are fortunate to have to spend only a very small portion of their disposable income on food – somewhere in the 10% range. Is it smart to save money on such a small portion of your budget that impacts your health so greatly? Do you buy the cheapest car available? Do you buy the cheapest appliance you can find? Do you only frequent the cheapest restaurants in your hometown? Do you only employ the lowest bidder for your lawn service, A/C repair, home improvements, etc.? Does your home have the cheapest faucets, windows, insulation, light fixtures, and so on? Do you watch TV on the cheapest set you could find? Do you buy the cheapest clothes you can find anywhere? Do you entrust your car to the cheapest mechanic in town? I think the answer is "no, of course not" in most, if not all cases. And you shouldn't settle for the cheapest source of calories either.

You are worth more than the cheapest food! You want "value for money" however, so why not apply that thinking to what you put into the only body you'll ever have? Do you want to end up with preventable diseases that then have to be treated at the most expensive hospitals and health-care providers you can afford? The quality (and quantity – less of it) of foods you consume does make a difference in your health and quality of life – so don't cut corners when it comes to your health. That holds especially true when it comes to the health of children. What's unhealthy for adults is even more dangerous for young, growing bodies, so invest in their health with organic foods. And that may be in <u>your</u> best interest too: high pesticide levels in children have been linked to ADHD (attention-deficit hyperactivity disorder), among other things.

SURPRISE: the best (legal) athletic performance enhancers … also can do wonders for your overall health and well being

That's right, and they are 2 simple things anybody can do:

- Get enough sleep: don't worry about sleep interruptions – but **keep your bedroom dark** (and don't turn on the lights in the middle of the night, or surf the web if you can't sleep). Just as the brain needs sufficient sleep to consolidate newly acquired knowledge and skills, the body needs it also for optimal recovery from previous workouts. Exercising doesn't make you stronger or faster. The period of rest that follows does, and a chronic sleep deficit will reduce your performance gains or, worse yet, lead to setbacks, burnout or injury.

- Reduce your sugar intake: zero, or as close as you can get of the refined kind; minimal natural sugars from fruit, vegetables and other foods.

It's as simple as that. Sure there's tons of additional good advice (enough to write another book, so I'll keep this brief), some of which is contained in this book, but these are the 2 big ones. Of course the impact of these two strategies will be greatly enhanced if you keep your weight low (cutting out refined sugar will help), exercise regularly (cardio; resistance; core & stretching – you need'em all), eat right (quality & quantity of foods; timing; portion sizes; balanced; etc.), and cut your vices down (alcohol; tobacco; drugs; etc. – "zero" would be a good goal). And as for pure athletic performance, you still have to put the hard work in, and recovery (think "sleep", mainly) as well as optimal fueling are key.

Everybody loves a winner.
But in this case you'd be much better without it.

One could argue that the infamous "Western Diet" is the most successful diet in the world. It has become the "standard" way of eating in The United States and most highly industrialized countries, and now the Western Diet is conquering emerging economies and under-developed countries. And in lockstep, modern "civilization diseases" follow: obesity, heart disease, stroke, diabetes, cancer, and more. Study after study have shown that where indigenous diets have been abandoned in favor of cheap over-processed Western foods, the overall health of the population has declined (and waist lines increased), yet there does not appear to be a government in the world that has the backbone to call its country and the health of its citizens off limits to alien-to-the-human-body highly processed grains, refined sugars, cheap fats, and other chemical-laden, inferior food-like products. This failure of governments to protect its citizens, sadly, is pretty much out of your control. But you don't have to associate with that "winner". Instead you can stay in control of your health by controlling what goes into your body – minimally processed foods as part of a balanced diet, of local and/or organic origin whenever possible, like this book illustrates. It may take a little bit more effort to *swim upstream*, but "going with the flow" (of the mainstream Western Diet) will virtually guarantee that you'll wash up in that big C.D. (civilization disease) Pool. Get out while you can.

"But it tastes so good!"

Sure it does. Do you think millions of dollars spent on designing food-like products for the express purpose of being addictively good is wasted money? Ingenious food processors manage to take all the chicken leftovers that can't be served in any self-respecting kitchen and process it into a pink paste that looks like soft-serve ice cream. Disgusting you say? Think about that next time you dig into chicken nuggets that "taste so good". Obviously we cannot trust our taste buds to make healthy choices when confronted with over-processed foods that appeal to them (but we can trust them when the choices are healthy and wholesome).

What to do about it? It would help to ignore highly advertised food products altogether since advertising budgets quite often are indicative of inferior nutritional value. And you don't apply this "if it tastes or feels that good it must be O.K." theory to the rest of your life. Driving 100 mph hour might be an adrenaline rush, yet you restrain yourself, since it can have fatal consequences, or at least get you in serious trouble with the law. You don't binge-drink just because booze tastes so good. Most students on spring break wise up sooner or later to the fact that the hangovers (literally and figuratively) eventually aren't worth it. You don't give in to your sexual fantasies with your neighbor's spouse, since it tends to end up in major life complications, apart from the morality aspect. So why then shouldn't there be some self-restraint in a civilized society when it comes to eating? We are not talking severe hardships caused by chocolate withdrawal symptoms, but limiting the consumption of same to small quantities on an occasional basis. This brings up the next subject, namely …

"Am I supposed to never enjoy decadent treats ever again? Life isn't worth living without occasional indulgences."

I agree, and then some. You owe it to yourself to taste different foods, enjoy dinner with friends (which may not be always super healthy), explore cuisines when traveling overseas, and enjoy treats. Ditto for family get-togethers, and that traditional holiday meal of your choice that you remember fondly from childhood. But these "comfort foods" have to be accounted for.

Say you feel that you can't live without that piece of designer cake one day, or a handful of nuts between meals, never mind the extra 250 calories. No issues with that, but before you have that snack you should decide where you will cut back those 250 calories: a smaller piece of meat on your dinner plate? No rice pilaf, or considerably less? No wine with your dinner? Cut out the creamed corn? If your thinking goes along the lines of wanting to "eat your cake and have it too" (in other words have that treat in addition to everything else) you could be setting yourself up for some serious weight gain. Do the math: 250 extra calories a day (which would really only be a small piece of cake, and smaller than most portion sizes these days), if added every day ("come on, live a little") would add up to 91,250 calories a year! That could translate to a whopping 26 lbs. weight gain per year! Obviously that's not a sustainable strategy, even when you don't consume "surplus" calories every day. Just adding 250 calories once a week could add nearly 4 lbs. a year, which will add up quickly too. My advice: go ahead and splurge – but cut out an equivalent number of calories that same day. Or expend *an additional* 250 calories that day, any which way you choose.

"I don't want to know what's in .... [you name it – hot dogs, burgers, donuts, etc.]"

How curious. Would you buy a used car if the dealer told you that "you really don't want to know the collision and repair history of this car"? Would you be O.K. if the plant manager of the nearby chemical plant assured you that their products, emissions, waste products, etc. are perfectly safe, and "you really don't want to know the details, trust us"? You may not ask for an ingredient list of a particular dish at a restaurant, but if the owners flat out refused to furnish that information would you be O.K. with that, since ... you really rather not know anyway?

Certainly, you can make the conscious decision to accept genetically modified foods and the meat of cloned animals, unwise as that may be, but wouldn't you at least like to know about it? Most of us are repulsed by the thought of eating bloated livers of force-fed geese, but have no qualms about ignoring cruel and inhumane treatment of calves or other livestock, or the chemicals in the food chain that "we'd rather not know about". Thinking of these and many other examples, maybe you would agree that we should know a few things about the foods we put into the only bodies we'll ever have, for our immediate and long-term health, and that adopting the ostrich philosophy when it comes to food is not in our best interests. I am not suggesting that you launch exhaustive investigative research into any and all foods and food manufacturers' products and practices, but ignoring the readily available body of knowledge about questionable foods is obviously not the answer. When in doubt, ask questions, check the internet, or listen to people knowledgeable in those subjects, since what you don't know could very well hurt you.

Eat only when you are hungry, or eat before you get hungry?

"YES"

In other words it depends, and both scenarios can be right. Waiting with your next meal or snack until you feel hungry works if you recognize the subtle symptoms of hunger early (most people don't) and if you have good food choices nearby (now and later), in portion sizes that are small or you can control. This approach will help avoid eating when your body really doesn't need any calories yet. On the other hand if your window of opportunity closes on you (like lunch hour in a plant) and you know you won't make it until you have access to good food choices until after work, it may be best to still have that meal or snack, but reduce portion size. Carrying a healthy snack with you is always a good insurance policy. A banana or a healthy energy bar (Lärabar™ comes to mind) or similar items travel well and keep you away from less-than-healthy choices at vending machines.

FOOD RANKINGS – USE WITH CAUTION:

Reducing a food's value to a single number is problematic at best, counter-productive at worst. It can still be a useful tool, however, if used properly, keeping in mind that absolute food ranking systems do not represent the absolute truth. Eating only "100"-rated foods will not make you healthier than eating a mix of differently-valued items, across categories. The opposite is true, since this simplistic approach would result in a seriously imbalanced diet. And a "32"-rated item is not necessarily unhealthier for you at any given time than an item rated a "71".

The usefulness of the 1-100 points ranking system lies more in providing **comparative data** within food groups, taking note of 'trends', accentuating differences in seemingly identical foods, making smart choices, and "off-setting" low-ranked foods that still have desirable nutritional qualities with higher ranked items.

For example:

- Note how the lowest ranked seafood (with the exception of lobster) is ranked higher – by a wide margin - than the highest ranked meat or poultry. And, when average values are compared it's not even close – seafood wins by a huge margin. This is a message worth listening to.

- Note how processed food is ranked significantly lower than its more wholesome sibling. Compare white rice numbers vs. brown rice numbers, instant oatmeal vs. old-fashioned oatmeal, and orange juice vs. whole oranges. More messages. And it takes the near-sainthood goodness out of apple pie. Sink your teeth into a crisp organic apple instead.

- Note how the "90 & above" category is the exclusive domain of vegetables and fruits? Another major message – but not to be interpreted as eating those foods in excess without balancing them with proteins, other carbs, fiber, and healthy oils.

- You can expect higher ratings from nuts or seeds than from their extracted oils, but they would still rank higher than vegetable oils. Therefore it's a safe bet to <u>add</u> fewer fat calories to your foods in the form of oils and fats, but instead make room for even healthier, nutrition-packed nuts, seeds, avocadoes, olives, etc. And some good protein sources have healthy fat profiles – think fish.

- Ditto for natural peanut butter consisting of just that – peanuts (and maybe a little bit of salt) vs. supermarket peanut butters loaded with hydrogenated fats, sugar, sodium, preservatives, etc.

- Can't live without certain 'bottom feeders' on the nutritional value chart? At the very least combine them with highly ranked items, to avoid '<u>suicide meals</u>' like fried c.c. eggs, bacon, and a plain bagel for breakfast, a salami on white bread sandwich for lunch, and pork ribs for dinner. Side of cola anyone?

- Also pay attention to the **high pesticide loads** of some vegetables and fruit. Some of these poisons <u>cannot</u> be removed by cleaning since they have penetrated the skin. However, all raw foods that are eaten with the peel should be thoroughly washed prior to consumption. After all you don't want to get sick from easily removed surface contaminants. Spray with a 50:50 mix of <u>water and vinegar</u> which will kill a lot more germs (and remove at least some pesticide residues) than water alone. "Scrub-or-rub" (or soak), as appropriate, then rinse with water and you are good to go. But it is not a "get out of [the pesticide] jail" free card! The worst offenders (sometimes referred to as the Dirty Dozen) have been identified in the list. To keep things confusing, this list (of high pesticide-load vegetables and fruits) changes every so often! Your best defense against the worst offenders: stay informed which foods are on the "least wanted" list of high pesticide loads, buy organic instead, avoid altogether, or eat rarely, and give them the vinegar-water treatment. Remember: this is not a case of "real men don't wash their fruit" since "real men", too, are powerless against carcinogens and surface contaminants, not to mention obesogens in pesticides, which can promote weight gain.

- Sadly lacking in this first attempt of over- simplifying food choices is the value of far superior wild-caught fish vs. farm-raised (worst with imported shellfish, but PCBs in farmed salmon are no trivial matter either), organic meats & pasture-raised poultry (and eggs!) vs. commercial beef and c.c. chickens & eggs, and fresh local farmers market–type foods vs. big carbon footprint produce from mega mono cultures, grown in depleted soils (if it isn't in the soil, it sure isn't in the produce grown in it either).

- And speaking of shellfish … this is where the old "buy domestic" recommendation may just be the best advice. While wild-caught seafood is nearly always preferable, special mention of the treatment of imported shrimp in particular is in order. Once a highly prized – and priced high – luxury, the ever-increasing demand for shrimp has resulted in the creation of untold unsanitary fish farms overseas (and here too). With increased supply to meet growing demand, prices have dropped and shrimp farmers try to squeeze every penny of profit out of their haul. Hence, no one should be surprised to learn that shrimp are crowded into ponds which are often filled with mud and banned-in-the-US chemicals, pesticides, antibiotics, disinfectants, sulfites and excrement. The quality of feed is in line with profit expectations (remember "buy low – sell high"), sanitary conditions can be appalling, and strict handling criteria are nearly impossible to adhere to (think long drives on un-refrigerated trucks from fish farms to processing plants in tropical countries). Chances are that whatever ice has been added to the dirty mess of shrimp on any given truck has melted long before the destination has been reached.

Then there are chlorine baths, the addition of sodium tripolyphosphates (to plump up the shrimp) and general filth to contend with. Surely the FDA is on top of this to protect us, right? Well, yes, in a typical government kind-of way. Approximately half (!) of inspected shipments are detained for various rule violations, salmonella and 'filth' included (yeah – the system works!), but since less than 2% of shipments are inspected you can calculate the odds of those yummy shrimp on your dinner plate having a clean bill of health (oh no - the system is broken!). Can't live without 'em? Sure you can, but if you "must" have them, at least buy them from your local supermarket or fishmonger clearly labeled "US Origin" or other, verifiable "responsible farming" claims. All bets are off with regards to what ends up on restaurant menus ("Would you like xenoestrogens with those shrimp?"), but beware that 90% or so of shrimp consumed in the US arrived here with a passport – another reason to "dine in" and know what's on your plate.

More words of caution: some foods on the Food Ratings spreadsheet get 'penalized' for one aspect (high fat, or salt, or sugar content typically) and should not necessarily be avoided. On the other hands some foods seem to be over-rated. See my (subjective) "remarks" next to the item in question, and then form your own opinion. Also note that the ratings are still of a very general nature, and don't cover a lot of foods yet. I suspect that the "interested parties" (when in doubt follow the money …) are still trying to gauge the impact this system will have on their (highly processed) offerings and their all-important bottom-line. It should be interesting to see what the final "product" (list) will look like – and don't bet the farm that there will even be one. Let's just say that "they" have been talking about this ranking system since 2008 …

SEAFOOD	SCORE	REMARKS
Salmon	87	
Tuna, Fresh	n.a.	
Halibut	82	Fish - the champion of high protein foods.
Cod	82	**Wild-caught is superior!**
Tilapia	82	(Some "responsibly farmed" seafood may be acceptable, but research of such
Snapper	82	fish farms is highly recommended. Read the facts on www.greenpeace.org in
Catfish	81	the article Aquaculture_Industry_01.pdf)
Oysters	81	
Swordfish	81	
Prawns	75	(If you knew how they are raised …..)
Shrimp	75	Avoid farm-raised, especially imported!
Clams	71	Log on to www.montereybayaquarium.org/cr/SeafoodWatch) for vital info. Also high in cholesterol, regardless of origin!
Tuna (canned)	67	
Scallops	51	Still better than best non-seafood protein choice
Lobster	36	Lowest ranked seafood - and that's *before* the butter

VEGETABLES & FRUIT	SCORE	REMARKS
Apricots	100	
Peaches	n.a.	**High pesticide load!!! Go for organic!!!**
Nectarines	n.a.	High pesticide load!! Go for organic!!
Asparagus	100	"Conventional-grown" usually safe
Beans (yellow and green)	100	
Blueberries	100	High pesticide load!! Go for organic!!
Broccoli	100	"Conventional-grown" usually safe
Cabbage	100	"Conventional-grown" usually safe
Cauliflower	100	
Kiwi	100	"Conventional-grown" usually safe
Lettuce (Green Leaf, Red Leaf & Romaine)	100	
Mustard Greens	100	
Okra	100	
Orange	100	"Conventional-grown" usually safe
Kale & Collard Greens	n.a.	High pesticide load! Go for organic!
Spinach	100	High pesticide load!! Go for organic!!
Strawberries	100	**High pesticide load!!! Go for organic!!!**
Cherries	n.a.	High pesticide load! Go for organic!
Turnip	100	
Carrots	99	
Grapefruit	99	"Conventional-grown" usually safe

Pineapple	99	"Conventional-grown" usually safe
Plums	99	
Radish	99	"Conventional-grown" usually safe
Bell Peppers	n.a.	High pesticide load!! Go for organic!!
Mushrooms	n.a.	"Conventional-grown" usually safe
Summer Squash	98	
Sweet potatoes; yams	96	
Apple	96	**High pesticide load!!! Go for organic!!!**
Pears	n.a.	
Green Cabbage	96	
Tomato	96	
Clementine	94	
Watermelon	94	"Conventional-grown" usually safe
Papaya	n.a.	"Conventional-grown" usually safe
Mango	93	"Conventional-grown" usually safe
Potatoes	93	High pesticide load! Go for organic!
Garlic	n.a.	
Onions	93	"Conventional-grown" usually safe
Tangerines	93	"Conventional-grown" usually safe
Bananas	91	"Conventional-grown" usually safe
Corn	91	
Fresh Figs	91	
Grapes	91	High pesticide load for imported grapes! Go for organic - or at least U.S.-grown!
Honeydew Melon	91	
Rhubarb	91	
Cranberries	n.a.	"Conventional-grown" usually safe
Eggplant	n.a.	"Conventional-grown" usually safe
Avocado	89	
Blackberries	83	
Raspberries	83	
Arugula	82	
Iceberg Lettuce	82	Over-rated! Go for field greens & spinach instead
Bok Choy	81	
Passion Fruit	78	
Celery	n.a.	**High pesticide load!!! Go for organic!!!**
Prunes	45	Nutritional powerhouse, but eat sparingly or suffer the consequences
Orange Juice	39	Use only 100% juice, then dilute with water to reduce sugar 'hit'
Dried Apples	34	O.K. if you can find without added sugar
Tomato Juice	32	Sodium bomb - go for whole tomatoes instead, or at least low-sodium version
Raisins	26	High sugar - but good nutritional value
Olives	24	Think healthy Greeks - but watch sodium intake

Coconut	24	Eat fresh young coconut meat instead
Sauerkraut	13	Fermented food with beneficial qualities; eat in moderation due to high sodium content
Apple Pie	2	Mom is still O.K. though

MEAT & POULTRY	SCORE	REMARKS
Turkey Breast (skinless)	48	Over-rated! Consider hormone content, drugs, chemicals, low-grade feed, unsanitary conditions and processing. Organic and pasture-raised O.K. however.
NY Strip Steak	44	Comes with a lot of baggage: saturated fats, cholesterol, plus poultry-type (mega-farm) issues too.
Chicken Breast (skinless)	39	Over-rated! Consider hormone content, drugs, chemicals, low-grade feed, unsanitary conditions and processing. Organic and pasture-raised O.K. however.
Pork Tenderloin	35	The "other white meat"? In your (advertising) dreams. There are (much) better animal-protein choices out there
Bottom Round Roast (Beef)	34	Comes with a lot of baggage: saturated fats, cholesterol, plus poultry-type (mega-farm) issues too.
Flank Steak (Beef)	34	Comes with a lot of baggage: saturated fats, cholesterol, plus poultry-type (mega-farm) issues too.
Turkey Breast	31	Over-rated! Consider hormone content, drugs, chemicals, low-grade feed, unsanitary conditions and processing. Organic and pasture-raised O.K. however.
Veal Chop	31	Raising calves takes animal cruelty to uncharted depths; organic farm-raised or bust!
Veal Leg Cutlet	31	Raising calves takes animal cruelty to uncharted depths; organic farm-raised or bust!
Beef Tenderloin	30	Comes with a lot of baggage: saturated fats, cholesterol, plus poultry-type (mega-farm) issues too.
Chicken Drumstick	30	Over-rated! Consider hormone content, drugs, chemicals, low-grade feed, unsanitary conditions and processing. Organic and pasture-raised O.K. however.
Ground Sirloin (Beef – 90/10)	30	Comes with a lot of baggage: saturated fats, cholesterol, plus poultry-type (mega-farm) issues too.
Pork Chop (boneless center cut)	28	The "other white meat"? In your (advertising) dreams. There are (much) better animal-protein choices out there
Chicken Wings	28	Over-rated! Consider hormone content, drugs, chemicals, low-grade feed, unsanitary conditions and processing. Organic and pasture-raised O.K. however. Plus, mostly skin, the unhealthiest part.
Ground Round (Beef - 85/15)	28	Comes with a lot of baggage: saturated fats, cholesterol, plus poultry-type (mega-farm) issues too.
Lamb Chops (loin)	28	Fewer mega-farm issues make this a better red meat choice than beef; organic is best
Leg of Lamb	28	Fewer mega-farm issues make this a better red meat choice than beef; organic is best
Ham (whole)	27	The "other white meat"? In your (advertising) dreams. There are (much) better animal-protein choices out there

Ground Chuck (Beef – 80/20)	26	Comes with a lot of baggage: saturated fats, cholesterol, plus poultry-type (mega-farm) issues too.
Pork Ribs, Country Style	25	The "other white meat"? In your (advertising) dreams. There are (much) better animal-protein choices out there
Beef Spareribs	24	Comes with a lot of baggage: saturated fats, cholesterol, plus poultry-type (mega-farm) issues too.
Pork Baby Back Ribs	24	The "other white meat"? In your (advertising) dreams. There are (much) better animal-protein choices out there
Fried Egg	18	How to destroy the highest quality animal protein. Go for boiled eggs instead (pasture raised)
Bacon	13	Fat & Cholesterol City: friends don't let friends eat bacon
Salami	7	Other processed sausages even worse?

GRAINS, NUTS, LEGUMES	SCORE	REMARKS
Old-fashioned oatmeal	88	"Best in Class?" - but load up with sugar and see score plummet
Walnuts		Lowers LDL **and** raises HDL. Walnuts for sainthood?
Almonds (raw)	82	
Pecans (raw)	82	
Brown Rice	82	**Best grain choice**
Silk® Light Soymilk	82	Allergic to soy? Try rice, almond or oat 'milks'
Couscous	72	Potential Wheat Allergy! Go for whole grain variety.
Pistachios (raw)	70	
Popcorn (plain)	69	"Plain" means no butter, no salt, no caramel
Instant Oatmeal	61	Go for old-fashioned - it doesn't take much longer to prepare and is hugely better for you
White Rice	57	AVOID: anything white rice can do, brown rice can do better. Tastes better too.
Lentils	n.a.	Most under-rated legume?
Kidney Beans	53	
Peas (canned)	49	Buy fresh or frozen instead
Whole Wheat Bread	30	Don't settle for "faux" WWB in supermarket bread aisle
Bagel	23	Potential Wheat Allergy AND Gluten Alert!
Peanut Butter (commercial)	23	Go for "real" PNB instead: stir once - enjoy for a long time. Refrigerate to keep oil from separating. You'll never go back to "Skip-It" commercial brands
Pretzels	11	Has image of 'healthy' snack - compared to what?
White Bread	9	Compare to brown rice and blanch … and never buy again
Saltine Crackers	2	Is anybody actually eating these?

196

ALKALINE vs. ACIDIC FOODS

The subject of food alkalinity vs. acidity appears to be a nutritional stealth topic which rarely gets any attention. This, despite the fact that it is universally accepted that consuming a diet heavily weighted in acid-forming foods is considered highly unhealthy. Ignore this subject at your own risk. An incomplete list of health problems that can be attributed to being over-acidic would include:

- Mineral imbalance: the body may "steal" alkalizing minerals from the body to keep the blood pH out of the acid range. A magnesium deficiency brought on (or made worse) by an over-acidic body is of particular concern. This situation can lead to reductions in bone density and an irregular heart beat, for example.
- Arthritic & rheumatoid diseases
- Fatigue
- Poor digestion – think diarrhea or constipation. This internal "self-poisoning" can lead to a host of more serious health problems!
- Many diseases thrive in an acid environment
- Heart burn, feeling bloated
- Insomnia
- Water retention
- Headaches

One reason for this issue being largely ignored is that it's complicated, poorly researched and understood, and no universally accepted guidelines are out there.

For one, there are few black and white areas, just lots of grays: not all acidic foods are 'evil', and solely consuming alkalizing foods is not a healthy way to live either. And the body's pH level is also affected by stress, physical activity, lifestyle, and other factors. There is not even universal consensus as to which foods are alkalizing and which are acid-forming. I have seen chocolate listed as alkalizing in some charts, but acid-forming in others. Ditto for natural (unsweetened) fruit juices. Take your pick? Even healthy vegetables, typically considered alkaline-forming, are sometimes rated differently, based on when they are grown, in what soil, and even in what direction relative to the earth axis! Don't expect for 'common sense' to help you make smart choices either: some clearly acidic foods such as citrus fruit actually have an alkalizing effect on the body once metabolized. Enough already, no?

So what to make of all this confusion, since *ignoring* it is not the answer? Use the attached (incomplete) list with these general guidelines:

- Use it wisely to <u>balance</u> acidic food intake with an adequate intake of alkalizing foods. Remember that many highly acid-forming foods are not "evil", but should be part of a healthy diet and should not be excluded. <u>It's all about balance.</u>

- When in doubt, err on the side of alkalizing foods, but never exclusively so.

- As a general guideline keep in mind that most meats, (including otherwise healthy) fish, eggs and grains, as well as most highly processed foods (which should be avoided for many other reasons) are acid forming, while most vegetables and fruit are alkalizing. Yet another reason to "eat your vegetables" like your mother told you – developing osteoporosis in what should be your prime years is neither fun nor cool.

- Consider adding highly alkaline seaweed to your diet. Not an easy sell that, but trust me – seaweed doesn't have to be that "slimy green vegetable". How would you explain the popularity of sushi restaurants worldwide? Last time I checked most California, tuna & salmon rolls were wrapped in seaweed. And you could always visit the nearest Oriental supermarket for <u>delicious seaweed snacks</u>. But examine the label closely – many of these products contain MSG, or sugar, or palm oil – or all three!

- Balance is the key, but why make it harder on yourself than you have to. Limiting highly acidic foods means you have to eat a lot less seaweed …. or other foods not high on your "like" list.

Acidic heavyweights to avoid: pork, veal, beef, liquor, beer, and sweetened fruit juices (or worse yet – "juice drinks"), to name only the worst offenders. There are better protein choices out there, and many healthy beverage alternatives.

Instead go for these …

Highly alkaline foods: most sprouts (soy, radish, etc), various grasses (wheat grass juice, alfalfa, barley), root vegetables in general, radishes in particular (black is best – if you can find it), the under-rated cucumber (an alkaline powerhouse) and aforementioned seaweed.

Alkaline vs. Acidic Foods

Highly Alkaline Foods - <u>eat often</u>	Comments
(Bolded Items are best)	
Degree of alkalinity (highest to lowest)	
Vegetables	
Wheat Grass +33.8	
Cucumber, Fresh +31.5	User-friendly: load up!
Soy Sprouts +29.5	Widely available, cheap, tasty - what's not to like?
Alfalfa Grass +29.3	Great in tossed salads
Sprouted Chia Seeds +28.5	
Sprouted Radish Seeds +28.4	
Barley Grass +28.1	
Kamut Grass +27.6	
Cayenne Pepper +18.8	
Endive, Fresh +14.5	
Celery +13.3	
Garlic +13.2	
Sorrel +11.5	
French Cut Green Beans +11.2	
Spinach, March Harvest +8.0	
Chives +8.3	
Watercress +7.7	
Leeks +7.2	
Red Cabbage +6.3	
Rhubarb +6.3	
Zucchini +5.7	
Peas, Fresh +5.1	
Savoy Cabbage +4.5	
White Cabbage +3.3	
Cauliflower +3.1	
Onion +3.0	
Green Cabbage	
Lettuce +2.2	Except iceberg lettuce
Asparagus +1.3	
Brussels Sprouts +0.5 Peas +0.5	

Root Vegetables	
Black Radish +39.4	
Red Radish +16.7	
Beet +11.3	
Carrot +9.5	
Turnip +8.0	
Horseradish +6.8	
Kohlrabi +5.1	
Rutabaga +3.1	
White Radish (Daikon) +3.1	
Potatoes +2.0	
Fruits	
Avocado +15.6	Yes, it's a fruit …
Tomato +13.6	That one too …
Fresh Lemon +9.9	
Limes +8.3	
Cherry, Sour +3.5	
Coconut, Fresh +0.5	
Unsweetened Fruit Juices, deleted with water 50:50	
Figs (dried & fresh)	
Organic Legumes	
Soy Lecithin +38.0	In moderation
Soy Nuts +26.5	In moderation
Cooked Ground Soy Beans +12.8	In moderation
Soybeans, Fresh +12.2	In moderation
White Beans (Navy Beans) +12.1	
Lima Beans +12.0	
Tofu +3.2	Highest quality plant proteins
Tempeh +3.1	
Soy Flour +2.5	In moderation
Lentils +0.6	

Nuts	
Almonds +3.6	
Brazil Nuts +0.5	
Seeds	
Pumpkin Seeds +5.6	
Sunflower Seeds +5.4	
Caraway Seeds +2.3	
Fennel Seeds +1.3	
Flax Seeds +1.3	
Cumin Seeds +1.1	
Sesame Seeds +0.5	
Fats (Fresh, Cold-Pressed Oils)	
Fish Oils +4.7	**Pure cod-liver oil** is best; fish pills good too
Evening Primrose Oil +4.1	
Flax Seed Oil +3.5	**Filtered** oil eliminates bitter taste
Borage Oil +3.2	
Olive Oil +1.0	The Gold Standard?
Organic Grains	
Buckwheat +0.5	
Spelt +0.5	It's still wheat
Herbs & Spices, etc.	
Chili Pepper	
Cinnamon	
Curry	
Ginger	
Herbs (all)	
Miso	
Sea Salt	Best Bet: REDMOND™ Real Salt
Stevia	No side effects, no chemicals, no calories
Tamari	
Turmeric	The Indian miracle spice - combine w. black pepper for best absorption

Consume in moderation	Comments
(Best to least within food group)	
Fruits	**All good - but balance with more vegetable servings**
Watermelon -1.0	
Grapefruit -1.7	
Red Currant -2.4	
Cantaloupe -2.5	
Cherry, Sweet -3.6	
Date -4.7	
Italian Plum -4.9	
Yellow Plum -4.9	
Raspberry -5.1	
Blueberry -5.3	
Strawberry -5.4	
Black Currant -6.1	
Cranberry -7.0	
Grape -7.6	
Gooseberry -7.7	
Currant -8.2	
Tangerine -8.5	
Mango -8.7	
Orange -9.2	
Papaya -9.4	
Apricot -9.5	
Peach -9.7	
Pear -9.9	
Banana -10.1	
Mandarin Orange -11.5	
Pineapple -12.6	
Rose Hips -15.5	

Grains	
Wheat -10.1	**Avoid**
Brown Rice -12.5	Best grain overall
White Rice	**Avoid**
Nuts	
Hazelnuts -2.0	
Macadamia Nuts -3.2	
Walnuts -8.0	Nutritional Powerhouse!
Fish	
Fresh Water Fish -11.8	Wild-caught only
Fats	
Peanut Oil	"Good Oil" (Neutral)
Macadamia Nut Oil	
Walnut Oil	
Almond Oil	
Canola Oil	
Coconut Milk -1.5	Small quantities O.K., without added sugar
Sunflower Oil -6.7	

Highly Acidic Food - avoid or limit consumption	Comments
(Worst to least within food group - avoid bolded items)	
Degree of acidity (highest to lowest)	
Meat, Poultry, And Fish	
Pork -38.0	Avoid
Veal -35.0	Avoid
Beef -34.5	Avoid
Chicken (to -22) -18.0	In moderation - pasture raised only!
Eggs (to -22)	Pasture-raised only!
Ocean Fish -20.0	All good if wild-caught and balanced w. alkaline vegetables
Oysters -5.0	O.K. in moderation
Organ Meats -3.0	O.K. in moderation
Processed Grains	
White Bread & white pasta -10.0	Avoid all!
Whole-Meal Bread -6.5	Go gluten-free: brown rice bread, millet bread.
Whole-Grain Bread -4.5	
Rye Bread -2.5	
Nuts	
Pistachios -16.6	O.K. in moderation
Cashews -9.3	O.K. in moderation
Legumes	
Peanuts -12.8	O.K. in moderation
Fats	
Cottonseed Oil	**Don't. Go. There.**
Margarine -7.5	**Don't go there**
Corn Oil -6.5	Don't go there
Butter -3.9	Use rarely or replace with "Earth Balance"

Sweeteners	
Corn Syrup / High-Fructose Corn Syrup	Off the charts: don't go there
White Sugar -33.6	Don't go there
Artificial Sweeteners -26.5	Use as little as possible; **avoid aspartame**
Chocolate -24.6	100% cocoa O.K. in moderation
Dried Sugar Cane Juice -18.0	
Beet Sugar -15.1	
Molasses -14.6	You can - or should - live without these
Malt Sweetener -9.8	
Fructose -9.5	
Turbinado Sugar -9.5	
Barley Malt Syrup -9.3	
Brown Rice Syrup -8.7	"Least Bad", but will still rot your teeth out
Honey -7.6	
Maple Syrup	
(Find Stevia under alkaline herbs & spices)	
Condiments	
Vinegar -39.4	A little goes a long way
Soy Sauce -36.2	Buy low-sodium
Mustard -19.2	Golden-yellow has turmeric
Mayonnaise -12.5	Avoid: buy "Vegenaise" or "Nayonaise" instead
Ketchup -12.4	Avoid
Beverages	
Liquor -38.7	Nothing good about it
Tea (Black) -27.1	Decaf in moderation O.K.
Beer -26.8	No, it's not 'liquid bread'
Coffee -25.1	Decaf in moderation O.K.
Wine -16.4	It's not health food
Decaf Green Tea	**The good stuff**

Miscellaneous	
Processed Foods	Eliminate and feel better
Dairy Products	Eliminate and feel better
Canned Foods	Eliminate and feel better
Herbs & Spices, etc.	All good in moderation, except table salt
Black Pepper	
Carob	
Cocoa	
Nutmeg	
Soy Sauce	
Table Salt	**Avoid! Use sea salt instead**
Vanilla	
Yeast (Nutritional; Brewer's)	Good, but use in moderation

GLYCEMIC INDEX

Yet another way to categorize foods, complete with charts which aren't necessarily universally accepted and which don't specifically identify "good foods" vs. "bad foods" - an illusionary concept to begin with anyway.

The glycemic index simply scores each food (usually carbohydrates) by how quickly it is absorbed into the blood stream. Foods with a **high glycemic index** will give you that quick "hit", resulting in a quick blood sugar "high" (and increased insulin levels), soon to be followed by a corresponding "crash", or "low". Consume a lot of those over a long period of time and you are well on your way to type 2 DM (aka Adult Onset Diabetes). Also, think obesity, high blood pressure, a slew of cancers, and such. But, there is no need to eliminate these foods altogether, so read on.

A food associated with a **low glycemic index** will enter your blood stream slowly, over a much longer period of time, and without the sugar spikes. Bonus: you will not feel hungry for a longer time, avoiding overeating with all its disastrous health effects, and your body will secrete less insulin. If you concluded that most of your food should come from slowly absorbed "steady" low glycemic foods you are 100% correct. But it doesn't mean that all high G.I. foods are bad for you – they just serve a different purpose. Some of them are very nutritious and should be part of a healthy diet. For example, during and immediately after strenuous and/or long physical exertion, high G.I. foods will be absorbed quickly, and furnish 'energy on demand', usually with less stress on the digestive system. Think of Muslims who typically "break the fast" during Ramadan with dates – one of the highest G.I. foods known to mankind - even higher than plain sugar (!), but nutritionally far superior.

How best to use this list? You can't go wrong with low glycemic foods but whenever you consume healthy high glycemic foods (watermelons, dates, millet, parsnips, potatoes, etc.) do so in moderation and balance them with low-glycemic food choices. When in doubt, err on the side of 'lovely-low' glycemic foods.

This attached G.I. list is especially important for people who want to lose weight, since high G.I. foods can result in a wild roller-coaster ride of highs and lows (a very unhealthy condition), followed by cravings for more "hits". If that sounds like a sugar-dependency problem to you, you are 100% correct again, so staying with low G.I. foods is the smart choice. They <u>will</u> reduce your sugar cravings. However, like any food, you must wait for the 'slow train' to reach your brain cells to give you the "all full" signal (after approx. 25 minutes).

The worst high G.I. offenders that <u>will</u> wreck your health: all processed white flour and refined sugar products (90% of the bread aisle, cakes, pastries, donuts, etc.) as well as white rice and white rice products (sticky rice anyone?), pretzels, chips, French fries, mashed potatoes, etc. And of course all those sugary soft drinks that don't really qualify as "food", yet add an ever-increasing amount of calories to the American diet. Not worried yet? Maybe the popular saying in the medical community ***"Sugar Feeds Cancer"*** is scary enough for you. And since most high G.I. foods are loaded with sugar, they will enable you to forego bothersome tooth brushing at an early age – since you can soak your dentures overnight for easy cleaning instead. Give it some thought.

Also note how the refined version of the same basic food on the G.I. list compared to the whole, unrefined version (for example white bread vs. whole grain bread) invariably has higher G.I. <u>and</u> G.L. ratings. Not good. It pays to go with "whole" and minimally processed.

A WORD ABOUT GLYCEMIC LOAD

Now that you are more knowledgeable about the glycemic index concept, here is this confusing fact: **<u>Glycemic Load</u>** is really the more important number to consider when making food choices. This factor takes into account the <u>amount</u> of carbohydrates in a food, and is calculated by multiplying the G.I. by the amount of carbohydrates in a serving of food, then divided by 100. All of a sudden a high G.I. food that has low amounts of carbohydrates can have a very low glycemic load factor. Here's an example to illustrate that point: watermelon has a high G.I. of 72, and would appear to wreak havoc on your blood sugar levels (and, if eaten by itself in sufficient quantities will do so). But since a serving of watermelon only contains 6 grams of carbs, the G.L. per serving is a 'friendly' 4. (Still, make sure to have it as part of a real meal.) Conversely, foods with a medium G.I. factor can "get you" with a huge glycemic load impact (soft drinks, commercial cereals, candy bars, etc. – but even otherwise healthy brown rice). How about mashed potatoes or French fries? They are sky-high in both G.I. and G.L. - go for sweet potatoes instead, preferably plain (the best way by far), or mashed (O.K.), or fried (still better than French Fries).

NOTE: all values are approximate and can vary widely depending on type, brand, origin, season, etc. of foods. Diabetics, the obese, and people sensitive to blood sugar level fluctuations should consult with their health care professionals for dietary choices.

Beverages		Glycemic Index	Glycemic Load *	Comments
Tomato Juice	Low	38	4	
Apple juice	Low	40	12	
Soy milk	Low	40	6	Best beverage choice: R.O. filtered tap water (most
Carrot juice	Low	45	10	cities). Also good: decaf teas (white, green, herbal, fruit,
Pineapple juice	Low	46	12	roobois, oolong, black), fruit juices diluted w. water
Grapefruit juice	Low	48	9	
Orange juice	Medium	51	13	
Soft Drink (12oz)	Medium	68	23	**Negative health impact and high G.L. too: AVOID!**

Breads		Glycemic Index	Glycemic Load *	
Pumpernickel	Low	46	5	
Multi grain bread (whole grain)	Low	48	7	Stick with Ezekiel, Adventist, Mestemacher, Alvarado Bakery, Feldkamp or similar companies' products. Over 90% of supermarket "breads" are "nutrition-challenged"
Corn Tortilla	Medium	50	11	All it takes is corn, salt, lime
Chapatti (Indian wheat bread)	Medium	52	15	
Rye-flour bread (whole meal)	Medium	54	7	
Roti (wheat)	Medium	59	16	Some taste better than others - and all are nutritionally inferior. Ignore the hype and 'thin' health claims.
Baguette	Medium	60	10	
Croissant	Medium	67	17	
Bagel (Plain)	Medium	69	24	
White bread	High	73	10	
Waffles	High	76	10	Worst of the worst
Doughnut	High	76	15	

Dairy		Glycemic Index	Glycemic Load *	
Low-fat yogurt (artificially sweetened)	Low	15	2	
Milk, chocolate	Low	24	5	
Low- fat yogurt (sweetened)	Low	26	7	You can live without it
Milk, whole	Low	27	4	
Milk, Fat-free	Low	32	4	
Milk ,skimmed	Low	32	4	

Fruits		Glycemic Index	Glycemic Load *	**Great anytime, but more is not better, due to high sugar content of most fruits**
Tomatoes	Low	15	1	
Avocado	Low	15	4	
Grapefruit	Low	25	3	
Apricots (dried)	Low	31	10	
Apples	Low	38	6	
Pears	Low	38	4	
Plums	Low	38	4	
Strawberries	Low	40	1	

Peaches	Low	42	6	
Oranges	Low	44	5	
Grapes	Low	46	8	
Kiwi	Medium	52	6	
Bananas	Medium	54	14	
Mangoes	Medium	56	9	
Papaya	Medium	56	9	
Apricots	Medium	57	5	
Cherries	Medium	63	9	
Raisins	Medium	64	28	
Melon (Cantaloupe)	Medium	65	4	
Pineapple	Medium	66	12	
Watermelon	High	72	4	Great during or right after strenuous exercise!
Dates	High	103	18	

Grains		Glycemic Index	Glycemic Load *	
Pearl Barley	Low	25	10	
Rye	Low	34	13	
Wheat kernels	Low	41	14	
Rice, instant	Low	46	18	Gluten-free, but inferior to brown rice
Corn	Medium	53	15	Gluten-free
Oat Bran	Medium	54	3	
Rice, brown	Medium	55	18	**Gluten-free & preferred**
Rice, wild	Medium	57	18	Not really a grain, but gluten-free & nutritious
Oatmeal	Medium	58	16	
Rice, white	Medium	64	23	Gluten-free, but inferior to brown rice
Millet	High	65	22	Gluten-free
Barley, flakes	Medium	66	25	
Sticky Rice	High	88	25	Gluten-free, but inferior to brown rice

Legumes		Glycemic Index	Glycemic Load *	
Peanuts	Low	14	1	
Soya beans (boiled)	Low	16	1	
Lentils (red, boiled)	Low	26	5	
Kidney beans (boiled)	Low	29	7	
Lentils (green, boiled)	Low	29	5	
Chickpeas (canned)	Low	38	9	
Black-eyed peas	Low	41	11	**Low G.I. nutritional powerhouses!**
Baked beans (canned)	Low	48	9	
Peas	Low	48	3	
Kidney beans (canned)	Medium	52	9	
Lentils (green, canned)	Medium	52	9	
Broad beans	High	79		

Roots		Glycemic Index	Glycemic Load *	Best [nutritional] bang for the buck!
Yam	Medium	51	18	
Sweet potato	Medium	54	17	
Taro	Medium	54	4	
Potato (boiled)	Medium	56	12	
Beets	Medium	63	4	

Carrots	High	71	3	Low glycemic load makes this a healthy choice
French Fries	High	75	22	
Mashed Potatoes	High	83	20	
Potato, baked	High	85	26	"Baked" means "plain", not "loaded"
Parsnips	High	97	12	

Sugars & Sweeteners		Glycemic Index	Glycemic Load *	
Stevia	Low	0	0	Non-caloric gold standard - no known side effects
Xylitol	Low	8	1	Low-cal natural sugar alternative; use in moderation (laxative effects)
Fructose	Low	20	2	Low G.I. does **not** make it healthy - and High Fructose Corn Syrup is worse!
Jams and Jellies	Medium	54	8	Avoid, or use sugar-free, or w/o added sugar
Sucrose	Medium	65	6	Avoid
Honey	High	74	16	All natural product - but will rot your teeth out nevertheless
Glucose	High	96	10	Avoid

Vegetables		Glycemic Index	Glycemic Load *	Your body's best friends - all of them
Cabbage	Low	6		
Mushrooms	Low	10		
Brussels Sprouts	Low	15		
Artichoke	Low	15		
Asparagus	Low	15		
Broccoli	Low	15		
Cauliflower	Low	15		
Celery	Low	15		Not tested or well researched due to minimal glycemic loads of most vegetables; usually rated between 0-1. Yet another reason to load up on vegetables.
Cucumber	Low	15		
Eggplant	Low	15		
Green beans	Low	15		
Lettuce, all varieties	Low	15		
Bell Peppers	Low	15		
Snow peas	Low	15		
Spinach	Low	15		
Summer squash	Low	15		
Zucchini	Low	15		

Low G.I. = less than 50
Medium G.I. = 50 - 70
High G.I. = more than 70

Low G.L. = 10 or less
Medium G.L. = 11-19
High G.L. = 20 or more

* per serving

TAKE-HOME MESSAGES

There are none

<u>Therefore:</u>

1.   Read the whole book.
2.   Read it in sequence – this is not a mystery novel or a catalog where you'll flip to the pages that have the stuff that interests you most. All the information is structured such that you need to have a basic understanding of one chapter before you can fully appreciate the next chapter.
3.   There are no shortcuts: it has taken you a long time to get out of shape, and hastily skipping pages will not get you to your goal any faster.
4.   <u>This time, do it right.</u> There are many weight loss theories out there, some good, some bad, and some ridiculous. Chances are you have tried a few of them, all without long-term success, so maybe the time is right to *revolutionize* your approach. Give the Diet Revolution Now System 100% and <u>you **will** be successful.</u> The more dedication you bring to the table, the more attention you pay to all aspects, the more successful you will be.
5.   Looking for the miracle weight loss secret in this book? It's there - but it's not one single "thing", and certainly not a miracle pill. It's the whole system - and your dedication - that will make things happen for you.

Is this the first chapter you are reading? Bad boy (or girl)! Now go back to page one ... ☺

Here's the best way to use this book: read it once, "digest" it, make appropriate changes, and keep it handy for reference. <u>After a few days or weeks read it again,</u> this time with high-lighter in hand, and mark the critical-for-you parts. This 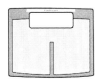 will re-enforce what you have learned already, help discover things that you missed the first time around, and then you'll have an even better reference book to go back to. Use it a lot, make notations, add comments or new diet findings, and make good use of the scale and the scale placemat - they can be your best friends and powerful allies.

---

* How to receive your placemat:

- Log on to www.dietrevolutionnow.com
- Submit proof of purchase of book

Placemat will be shipped anywhere in the Continental U.S. at no charge.

CPSIA information can be obtained at www.ICGtesting.com
Printed in the USA
LVOW060915220212

269891LV00001B/3/P